Cooking for Meniere's Relief

60 Flavorful, Low-Sodium Recipes to Ease Symptoms and Enhance Wellness

Anita F. MS, RDN. McCluskey

<u>Dedication</u>

To every hero with Meniere's disease, may this book bring comfort and guidance, and help you discover joy in nourishing yourself each day. And to my family and friends, for your endless love, patience, and encouragement— you are my foundation and my inspiration.

Contents

Chapter 5: Soothing Dinners for Relaxation and Relief

Chapter 6: Symptom-Soothing Snacks and Sides

6. Baked Kale Chips

7. Carrot and Celery Sticks with Herb Dip

8. Apple Slices with Almond Butter

9. Steamed Edamame with Lemon

10. Mixed Nuts and Seed Trail Mix

<u>Chapter 7:</u> Tasty Desserts Without Excess Salt or Sugar

1. Berry Chia Pudding

2. Fresh Fruit Salad with Lime Drizzle

3. Banana Nice Cream

4. Baked Apples with Cinnamon

5. Oatmeal Cookies with Dark Chocolate Chips

6. Coconut Mango Rice Pudding

7. Avocado Chocolate Mousse

8. No-Bake Almond Date Energy Bites

9. Poached Pears with Ginger Syrup

10. Raspberry Yogurt Parfait

<u>Chapter 8:</u> Hydration and Nourishing Beverages

1. Herbal Teas for Inner Ear Health

2. Low-Sugar Berry Smoothie

3. Electrolyte Balancing Infused Water

Conclusion

Understanding Meniere's Disease

Meniere's disease can feel like a sudden storm, bringing unanticipated disruptions, a sense of isolation, and challenging symptoms. But there is a path to calm within the chaos. **Joan Wilbert**, a sales receptionist, once battled constant dizziness and the looming threat of vertigo, which made everyday life difficult. By making small, impactful adjustments to her diet and lifestyle, *Joan* found balance and relief. Her journey—going from feeling limited by Meniere's to reclaiming control—inspired this book. With a structured meal plan and a renewed focus on self-care, *Joan* experienced reduced symptoms, steadier hearing, and a renewed vitality.

Cooking for Meniere's Relief was designed to help you, like Joan, find relief and discover how dietary changes can make a real difference. This collection of simple, low-sodium recipes, paired with practical guidance, aims to support you in managing symptoms, lowering the risk of flare-ups, and living confidently.

Our goal is to equip you with the knowledge, tools, and encouragement you need to move forward with optimism. You deserve mornings where you feel strong and prepared for whatever comes your way. Let this book become your companion, guiding you to a more vibrant life, where you feel supported, empowered, and capable. Together, we'll turn your kitchen into a haven of nourishment, comfort, and healing. With thoughtful choices, you can find calm amidst Meniere's and regain your peace of mind.

The Role of Diet in Managing Meniere's Symptoms

For individuals with Meniere's disease, diet plays a crucial role in symptom management. The foods you consume can greatly affect how often and intensely symptoms like vertigo, tinnitus, and imbalance occur. By thoughtfully adjusting her diet, Joan found that reducing high-sodium foods and including anti-inflammatory ingredients were key steps toward achieving greater stability and comfort.

This cookbook offers a variety of flavorful, low-sodium recipes specifically designed to support inner ear health. Each recipe is crafted to be easy to prepare while providing relief and maintaining delicious flavors. Alongside recipes, you'll find meal plans and lifestyle tips that go beyond nutrition—providing guidance on managing stress, staying active, and developing healthy habits to promote long-term wellness. Remember, even small changes can make a big difference, and you're not alone on this journey.

How to Use This Cookbook for Optimal Relief

Cooking for Meniere's Relief is more than just recipes; it's a well-rounded guide to integrating symptom-friendly meals into your daily routine. Start by exploring dishes that catch your interest, from breakfasts and lunches to dinners, snacks, and satisfying desserts. Each recipe is carefully crafted to be both beneficial for managing Meniere's and enjoyable to eat.

The included meal plans provide a weekly structure to help you minimize symptoms and find relief. Begin by swapping a few meals, then gradually transition to a full dietary approach over time. As Joan's experience shows, consistency is key to seeing results—every small dietary shift contributes to your journey toward comfort and balance. Embrace each step, celebrate your progress, and enjoy the rewarding process of nourishing your body.

With the support of this cookbook, you can enhance your wellbeing, reduce symptoms, and greet each day with new optimism. You deserve a life filled with stability, energy, and joy, and *Cooking for Meniere's Relief* is here to help you achieve that.

Chapter 1

Nutrition and Meniere's Disease

Key Nutritional Strategies for Symptom Management

Effectively managing Meniere's disease starts with understanding how essential nutrition is in controlling symptoms. Dietary adjustments can be one of the most powerful tools for easing symptoms. For Joan Wilbert, adopting a meal plan that prioritized low-sodium options, boosted hydration, and incorporated anti-inflammatory ingredients made a significant difference in her wellbeing. These core nutritional principles will guide you on your own path to finding relief from symptoms.

Low-Sodium Diet: A Key to Reducing Vertigo

A low-sodium diet is crucial for managing symptoms of Meniere's disease. High sodium intake can cause the body to retain fluid, increasing pressure in the inner ear and intensifying vertigo episodes. Reducing sodium helps balance fluid levels, directly alleviating these symptoms. Joan's story demonstrates this well: by cutting out processed foods and opting for fresh, whole ingredients, she saw a significant drop in the frequency and intensity of her vertigo.

This book offers low-sodium recipes that are full of flavor, so you won't need to compromise on taste. Using a variety of herbs, spices, and fresh ingredients, these dishes are crafted to support your health while delighting your palate.

The Importance of Hydration and Balanced Nutrients

Staying properly hydrated is also essential for managing Meniere's. Good hydration supports electrolyte balance and helps reduce fluid buildup, which can otherwise trigger symptoms. Simple habits like drinking water consistently and incorporating hydrating, nutrient-rich foods into your diet can promote stability and help prevent dehydration, a common factor that can worsen symptoms.

Alongside hydration, a balanced nutrient intake is key. Anti-inflammatory foods—such as leafy greens, berries, and omega-3 sources like flaxseeds—not only reduce inflammation but also support overall health, energy, and inner ear function. This book's recipes are rich in these nourishing ingredients, making it easy to focus on foods that benefit your body.

With these foundational steps, you're well on your way to effectively managing Meniere's symptoms. Like Joan, you can use nutrition to improve your wellbeing, reduce symptoms, and enhance your quality of life. As you explore each chapter, you'll gain the tools and confidence to take control of your health, one meal at a time

Chapter 2

Essential Ingredients for the Meniere's Diet

Effectively managing Meniere's disease starts with knowing which ingredients can support your body while easing symptoms. In this chapter, you'll explore key pantry staples, aromatic herbs and spices, and useful tips for choosing ingredients wisely. These elements will help you create meals that are not only delicious but also promote better health.

Pantry Staples for a Low-Sodium Kitchen

Creating a low-sodium kitchen doesn't mean sacrificing flavor or satisfaction. Here are some key pantry staples to keep on hand:

1. **Whole Grains:** Incorporate grains like brown rice, quinoa, farro, and oats for essential nutrients and fiber, which support digestive health and maintain energy levels.

2. **Legumes:** Beans, lentils, and chickpeas are rich in protein and fiber, helping you feel full and providing important nutrients.

3. **Nuts and Seeds:** Stock up on almonds, walnuts, chia seeds, and flaxseeds for healthy fats, fiber, and protein. They can enhance salads, smoothies, or snacks.

4. **Low-Sodium Broths:** Choose vegetable or chicken broth labeled as low sodium. These are great bases for soups, stews, and sauces without adding extra salt.

5. **Canned or Frozen Vegetables:** Opt for "no salt added" or "low sodium" options to save time while ensuring nutritious ingredients are always available.

6. **Whole-Grain Pasta:** Select whole-grain or legume-based pasta for more nutrients and fiber compared to traditional white pasta.

7. **Healthy Oils:** Use olive oil, avocado oil, or coconut oil for cooking and dressings to enhance flavors and provide healthy fats.

Herbs and Spices for Flavor Without Salt

Using herbs and spices to flavor your meals can greatly enhance their taste without the need for extra salt. Here are some essential options to stock in your kitchen:

1. **Garlic:** Fresh garlic or garlic powder adds a rich flavor to dishes while offering anti-inflammatory benefits.

2. **Ginger:** This warming spice is beneficial for digestion and nausea, making it ideal for managing Meniere's symptoms. Use it fresh in stir-fries or as a soothing tea.

3. **Turmeric:** Known for its anti-inflammatory properties, turmeric contributes an earthy flavor and beautiful color to soups and curries.

4. **Basil and Oregano:** These fresh or dried herbs elevate the taste of pasta dishes, salads, and marinades, adding a Mediterranean touch.

5. **Cilantro and Parsley:** Fresh herbs like cilantro and parsley can brighten meals, perfect for salads, salsas, or as a garnish.

6. **Cumin and Coriander:** These spices add warmth and depth to stews and curries, offering rich flavors without the need for salt.

7. **Lemon and Lime Juice:** The acidity from citrus can enhance flavors and provide a refreshing twist to dressings, marinades, and beverages.

Tips for Choosing the Right Ingredients

Making thoughtful ingredient selections can support your path to improved health. Here are some practical recommendations:

1. **<u>Read Labels:</u>** Always check food labels for sodium levels, aiming for products with 140 mg of sodium or less per serving.

2. **<u>Opt for Fresh:</u>** Whenever possible, select fresh produce over processed foods, as fresh fruits and vegetables are naturally low in sodium and packed with nutrients.

3. **<u>Buy Organic:</u>** Organic fruits and vegetables are often more nutritious and free from harmful pesticides, making them healthier options for your meals.

4. **<u>Shop Seasonally:</u>** Choosing seasonal produce usually means fresher, tastier, and often cheaper options. Visit local farmers' markets or grocery stores for the best selections.

5. **<u>Plan Your Meals:</u>** Planning meals in advance can help you make healthier choices and avoid the temptation of processed snacks or meals.

6. **<u>Experiment:</u>** Don't hesitate to try new ingredients or cooking techniques. Variety keeps meals exciting and prevents boredom.

By integrating these essential ingredients and tips into your cooking habits, you can create meals that are not only delicious but also supportive of your health and wellbeing. The upcoming chapters will feature a variety of recipes designed to nourish your body while helping you effectively manage Meniere's symptoms. Enjoy the exciting journey of discovering how flavorful and satisfying a low-sodium diet can be!

Chapter 3

Breakfast Recipes for a Strong Start to Your Day

Breakfast is widely considered the most important meal of the day, particularly for those managing Meniere's disease. Choosing nourishing, low-sodium options in the morning can have a profound impact on how you feel throughout the day. The recipes in this chapter are designed to be easy to prepare, satisfying, and nutritious, helping you begin your day with greater energy and a positive outlook.

Anti-Inflammatory Berry Smoothie Bowl

This colorful smoothie bowl is rich in antioxidants and anti-inflammatory components, making it an ideal way to begin your day. It's refreshing, flavorful, and can be personalized with various toppings.

Ingredients

- 1 cup frozen mixed berries (blueberries, strawberries, raspberries)
- 1 banana
- 1 cup unsweetened almond milk (or any plant-based milk)
- 1 tablespoon chia seeds
- 1 tablespoon almond butter
- Fresh berries and banana slices for topping
- Granola or nuts for added crunch (optional)

Step-by-Step Instructions

1. Combine the frozen mixed berries, banana, almond milk, chia seeds, and almond butter in a blender.
2. Blend on high until smooth and creamy.
3. Pour the smoothie into a bowl.
4. Top with fresh berries, banana slices, and optional granola or nuts.

Nutritional Information (per serving)

- Calories: 250
- Protein: 6g
- Carbohydrates: 40g
- Fiber: 8g
- Sugars: 15g
- Fat: 9g

Tips and Tricks

- For a thicker consistency, freeze the banana beforehand.
- Feel free to swap in different fruits like mango or spinach for added nutrients.

Quinoa Porridge with Fresh Berries

This warm quinoa porridge offers a comforting breakfast option packed with nutrients and lasting energy. As a complete protein, quinoa makes this dish both healthy and filling.

Ingredients

- 1 cup cooked quinoa
- 1 cup almond milk (or any plant-based milk)
- 1 teaspoon cinnamon

- 1 tablespoon maple syrup or honey (optional)
- 1/2 cup fresh berries (blueberries, strawberries, raspberries)
- Chopped nuts for topping (optional)

Step-by-Step Instructions

1. In a saucepan, mix cooked quinoa, almond milk, cinnamon, and maple syrup or honey.
2. Heat over medium, stirring occasionally until warmed through.
3. Serve in a bowl and top with fresh berries and nuts.

Nutritional Information (per serving)

- Calories: 220
- Protein: 8g
- Carbohydrates: 35g
- Fiber: 5g
- Sugars: 5g
- Fat: 7g

Tips and Tricks

- Prepare a batch of quinoa in advance for quick breakfast options during the week.
- Add a scoop of nut butter for extra protein.

Low-Sodium Vegetable Omelette

A vegetable omelette is a hearty breakfast option that is both satisfying and adaptable. This low-sodium version is filled with colorful veggies, offering vital nutrients to start your day right.

Ingredients

- 3 large egg whites
- 1/4 cup diced bell peppers
- 1/4 cup chopped spinach
- 1/4 cup diced tomatoes
- 1 tablespoon olive oil
- Fresh herbs for garnish (optional)

Step-by-Step Instructions

1. Whisk the egg whites in a bowl until slightly frothy.

2. Heat olive oil in a non-stick skillet over medium heat. Add bell peppers and tomatoes, sautéing until softened.

3. Stir in spinach and cook until wilted.

4. Pour the egg whites into the skillet, swirling to distribute the vegetables evenly.

5. Cook until the egg whites are set, fold the omelette in half, and serve.

Nutritional Information (per serving)

- Calories: 150
- Protein: 15g
- Carbohydrates: 6g
- Fiber: 2g
- Sugars: 2g
- Fat: 7g

Tips and Tricks

- Customize with additional vegetables like mushrooms or zucchini.
- Try different herbs and spices to enhance flavor without adding salt.

Banana Oat Pancakes with No-Added-Sugar Syrup

These fluffy pancakes, made with wholesome oats and ripe bananas, create a naturally sweet and nutritious breakfast suitable for any day.

Ingredients

- 1 cup rolled oats
- 1 ripe banana
- 1 cup almond milk
- 1 teaspoon baking powder
- 1 teaspoon vanilla extract
- Maple syrup or fruit puree for serving

Step-by-Step Instructions

1. Blend rolled oats, banana, almond milk, baking powder, and vanilla extract in a blender until smooth.
2. Preheat a non-stick skillet over medium heat.
3. Pour 1/4 cup of the batter onto the skillet for each pancake.
4. Cook until bubbles form on the surface, flip, and cook until golden brown.
5. Serve warm with maple syrup or fruit puree.

<u>**Nutritional Information (per serving, 2 pancakes)**</u>

- Calories: 220
- Protein: 5g
- Carbohydrates: 40g
- Fiber: 4g
- Sugars: 5g
- Fat: 4g

<u>**Tips and Tricks**</u>

- Add cinnamon or nutmeg to the batter for extra flavor.
- Make a larger batch and freeze leftover pancakes for quick breakfasts later.

<u>*Chia Seed Pudding with Almonds*</u>

Chia seed pudding is a delightful and nutritious breakfast option high in fiber and omega-3 fatty acids. It's simple to prepare and can be made the night before for a quick morning meal.

<u>**Ingredients**</u>

- 1/4 cup chia seeds

- 1 cup almond milk (or any plant-based milk)
- 1 tablespoon maple syrup (optional)
- 1/4 teaspoon vanilla extract
- Sliced almonds and fresh fruit for topping

Step-by-Step Instructions

1. In a bowl, whisk chia seeds, almond milk, maple syrup, and vanilla extract together.
2. Cover and refrigerate for at least 4 hours or overnight until thickened.
3. Serve topped with sliced almonds and fresh fruit.

Nutritional Information (per serving)

- Calories: 200
- Protein: 6g
- Carbohydrates: 18g
- Fiber: 12g
- Sugars: 5g
- Fat: 12g

Tips and Tricks

- Mix in flavors like cocoa powder or matcha for variety.

- Chia pudding also makes a healthy dessert option.

Avocado Toast with Lemon Zest

Avocado toast is a popular and nutritious breakfast choice that is quick to prepare. The creamy avocado offers healthy fats and fiber, making it a satisfying and tasty option.

Ingredients

- 1 ripe avocado
- 2 slices whole grain or gluten-free bread
- Lemon juice and zest
- Fresh herbs (such as cilantro or parsley) for garnish

Step-by-Step Instructions

1. Toast the bread slices until golden brown.
2. Mash the avocado in a bowl with lemon juice and zest.
3. Spread the avocado mixture onto the toasted bread.
4. Garnish with fresh herbs before serving.

<u>**Nutritional Information (per serving)**</u>

- Calories: 300
- Protein: 8g
- Carbohydrates: 40g
- Fiber: 12g
- Sugars: 2g
- Fat: 15g

<u>**Tips and Tricks**</u>

- Add sesame seeds or red pepper flakes for extra texture.
- Try different toppings like radishes or sliced tomatoes for a flavor boost.

<u>Overnight Oats with Apples and Cinnamon</u>

This easy, no-cook breakfast is both satisfying and nutritious. Full of fiber and whole grains, it keeps you full longer, while the apples and cinnamon provide a sweet touch without added sugar.

<u>**Ingredients**</u>

- 1 cup rolled oats

- 1 cup unsweetened almond milk (or your choice of non-dairy milk)
- 1 medium apple, chopped
- 1 teaspoon ground cinnamon
- 1 tablespoon chia seeds (optional)
- 1 tablespoon maple syrup (optional)
- ¼ cup chopped nuts (such as walnuts or almonds for extra protein)

Instructions

1. In a bowl, mix the rolled oats, almond milk, diced apple, cinnamon, chia seeds, and maple syrup if desired.

2. Stir well to ensure everything is combined.

3. Divide the mixture into jars or containers with lids.

4. Refrigerate overnight (or for at least 4 hours) to let the oats absorb the liquid and soften.

5. Before serving, give it a good stir and top with chopped nuts for added texture.

Nutritional Information (per serving)

- Calories: 290
- Protein: 8g

- Carbohydrates: 45g
- Fiber: 7g
- Sugars: 10g
- Fat: 8g

Tips and Tricks

- Personalize your overnight oats by adding different fruits like berries or bananas for extra flavor and nutrition.
- Prepare several jars at once for a quick breakfast option throughout the week.

Spinach and Mushroom Frittata

This delicious frittata is rich in protein and incorporates the health benefits of spinach and mushrooms, both known for their anti-inflammatory properties. It's an excellent choice for a leisurely breakfast or can be made ahead for the week.

Ingredients

- 6 large eggs
- 1 cup fresh spinach, chopped
- 1 cup mushrooms, sliced

- ½ cup low-fat milk (or a non-dairy alternative)
- ¼ teaspoon black pepper
- ¼ teaspoon garlic powder
- Olive oil for cooking

Instructions

1. Preheat the oven to 375°F (190°C).

2. In a skillet, heat a splash of olive oil over medium heat. Add the mushrooms and sauté until soft.

3. Stir in the chopped spinach and cook until wilted.

4. In a bowl, whisk together the eggs, milk, black pepper, and garlic powder.

5. Pour the egg mixture over the sautéed vegetables in the skillet. Let it cook for about 2-3 minutes until the edges start to set.

6. Transfer the skillet to the oven and bake for 15-20 minutes until the center is firm and the top is slightly golden.

7. Allow to cool for a few minutes before cutting into wedges.

<u>**Nutritional Information (per serving)**</u>

- Calories: 200
- Protein: 14g
- Carbohydrates: 3g
- Fiber: 1g
- Sugars: 1g
- Fat: 14g

<u>**Tips and Tricks**</u>

- Feel free to include additional vegetables like bell peppers or zucchini for more flavor and nutrients.
- This frittata can be stored in the refrigerator for up to three days, making it a convenient meal prep option.

<u>Buckwheat Pancakes with Blueberries</u>

These fluffy pancakes are made with nutritious buckwheat flour, which is naturally gluten-free and packed with protein and fiber. Topped with antioxidant-rich blueberries, they offer both great taste and health benefits.

Ingredients

- 1 cup buckwheat flour
- 1 tablespoon baking powder
- 1 tablespoon maple syrup (optional)
- 1 cup unsweetened almond milk (or any preferred non-dairy milk)
- 1 teaspoon vanilla extract
- ½ cup fresh or frozen blueberries

Instructions

1. In a bowl, combine buckwheat flour and baking powder.

2. In another bowl, whisk together almond milk, maple syrup, and vanilla extract.

3. Gradually mix the wet ingredients into the dry ingredients until just combined. Gently fold in the blueberries.

4. Heat a non-stick skillet or griddle over medium heat. Pour ¼ cup of the batter for each pancake onto the skillet.

5. Cook for 2-3 minutes until bubbles form on the surface, then flip and cook for another 1-2 minutes until golden brown.

6. Serve warm with a drizzle of maple syrup or a sprinkle of additional blueberries.

Nutritional Information (per serving)

- Calories: 180
- Protein: 5g
- Carbohydrates: 28g
- Fiber: 4g
- Sugars: 4g
- Fat: 5g

Tips and Tricks

- Try other fruits like sliced bananas or strawberries for different flavors.
- These pancakes freeze well, making them ideal for quick breakfasts later.

Ginger and Turmeric Smoothie

This colorful smoothie is filled with anti-inflammatory ingredients, blending the warming spices of ginger and turmeric with nutritious fruits. It's an excellent quick breakfast that energizes you for the day.

Ingredients

- 1 frozen banana
- 1 cup spinach
- ½ cup unsweetened almond milk (or your choice of non-dairy milk)
- 1 teaspoon fresh ginger, grated
- ½ teaspoon ground turmeric
- 1 tablespoon chia seeds
- ½ cup pineapple or mango chunks

Instructions

1. In a blender, combine the frozen banana, spinach, almond milk, ginger, turmeric, chia seeds, and pineapple or mango.
2. Blend until smooth, adding more almond milk if needed to achieve your desired consistency.
3. Pour into a glass and enjoy immediately.

Nutritional Information (per serving)

- Calories: 220
- Protein: 4g
- Carbohydrates: 46g
- Fiber: 7g
- Sugars: 20g

- Fat: 4g

<u>Tips and Tricks</u>

- For extra creaminess, add a scoop of avocado or use coconut yogurt.
- Adjust the sweetness with a little honey or agave if desired.

Chapter 4

Nourishing Lunches for Symptom Relief and Balance

Lunch plays a vital role in fueling your afternoon, helping you maintain energy and concentration throughout the day. For those managing Meniere's disease, a well-balanced lunch is key to stabilizing symptoms and promoting overall health. This chapter offers a selection of wholesome, flavorful recipes designed to ease symptoms while pleasing your palate.

These meals not only provide symptom relief but also supply essential nutrients to support your well-being. From fresh, vibrant salads to hearty wraps, each recipe is simple to prepare and bursting with flavor, ensuring you can enjoy lunch without stress.

With an emphasis on hydrating and low-sodium ingredients, these recipes are carefully crafted to reduce Meniere's-related issues while still being nutritious and delicious. Enjoy your lunches with peace of mind, knowing they are both healthful and satisfying.

Roasted Veggie and Quinoa Salad

This colorful salad brings together roasted vegetables and protein-rich quinoa, creating a filling and nutritious dish perfect for lunch. Its mix of textures and fresh flavors ensures a tasty and wholesome experience.

Ingredients

- 1 cup quinoa, rinsed
- 2 cups vegetable broth or water
- 1 zucchini, diced
- 1 bell pepper, diced
- 1 cup cherry tomatoes, halved
- 1 red onion, diced

- 2 tablespoons olive oil
- 1 teaspoon garlic powder
- 1 teaspoon dried oregano
- Salt and pepper to taste
- Fresh parsley, chopped (for garnish)

Step-by-Step Instructions

1. Preheat your oven to 400°F (200°C).

2. Toss the zucchini, bell pepper, cherry tomatoes, and red onion with olive oil, garlic powder, oregano, salt, and pepper in a large bowl.

3. Arrange the seasoned vegetables on a baking sheet and roast them in the oven for 20-25 minutes or until they are tender and slightly caramelized.

4. While the vegetables are roasting, bring the vegetable broth or water to a boil in a saucepan. Add the quinoa, reduce the heat to low, cover, and simmer until all the liquid is absorbed.

5. Fluff the cooked quinoa with a fork, then combine it with the roasted vegetables in a large bowl.

6. Serve warm, garnished with fresh parsley.

Nutritional Information per Serving

- Calories: 320
- Protein: 10g
- Carbohydrates: 45g
- Fat: 12g
- Fiber: 7g

Tips and Tricks

- Feel free to substitute seasonal vegetables for added variety.
- This salad can be prepared in advance and stored in the refrigerator for up to 3 days.
- For additional protein, consider adding grilled chicken or chickpeas.

Lemon Herb Chicken Wraps

These chicken wraps are a light yet satisfying option for lunch, packed with lean protein and fresh vegetables. The zesty lemon herb dressing adds brightness, making this dish both refreshing and nourishing.

Ingredients

- 2 whole grain tortillas

- 1 cup cooked chicken breast, sliced
- 1 cup mixed salad greens
- 1/2 cucumber, sliced
- 1/2 bell pepper, sliced
- 1/4 cup low-fat Greek yogurt
- 1 tablespoon lemon juice
- 1 teaspoon dried dill
- Salt and pepper to taste

Step-by-Step Instructions

1. In a small bowl, mix Greek yogurt, lemon juice, dill, salt, and pepper to make a dressing.
2. Spread a layer of the yogurt dressing on each whole grain tortilla.
3. Arrange the mixed greens, chicken, cucumber, and bell pepper on each tortilla.
4. Roll the tortillas tightly, folding in the sides to secure the filling.
5. Slice each wrap in half and serve immediately.

Nutritional Information per Serving

- Calories: 350
- Protein: 30g
- Carbohydrates: 40g

- Fat: 9g
- Fiber: 5g

Tips and Tricks

- Prep the chicken ahead of time for quick lunch assembly.
- For a vegetarian option, substitute chicken with hummus or baked tofu.

Low-Sodium Lentil Soup

This hearty lentil soup is perfect for a comforting lunch that's rich in fiber and protein while being easy on sodium. It's nourishing, flavorful, and will keep you feeling full and satisfied.

Ingredients

- 1 cup dried lentils, rinsed
- 1 medium onion, chopped
- 2 carrots, diced
- 2 celery stalks, diced
- 3 cloves garlic, minced
- 4 cups low-sodium vegetable broth
- 1 teaspoon ground cumin
- 1 teaspoon thyme

- Pepper to taste
- Fresh parsley for garnish

Step-by-Step Instructions

1. Sauté the onion, carrots, and celery in a large pot over medium heat until they soften.

2. Add the minced garlic and cook for an additional minute.

3. Stir in the lentils, vegetable broth, cumin, thyme, and pepper, and bring to a boil.

4. Reduce the heat and let it simmer uncovered until the lentils are tender.

5. Adjust seasoning if necessary, and serve garnished with fresh parsley.

Nutritional Information per Serving

- Calories: 240
- Protein: 18g
- Carbohydrates: 40g
- Fat: 1g
- Fiber: 15g

- Make a large batch to freeze for up to 3 months.
- Add extra veggies for enhanced nutrition and flavor.

Spinach and Chickpea Buddha Bowl

This vibrant Buddha bowl features a mix of grains, greens, and chickpeas, making it both nourishing and satisfying. The combination of fresh and cooked ingredients ensures a flavorful and balanced dish.

Ingredients

- 1 cup cooked brown rice or quinoa
- 1 cup fresh spinach
- 1 cup canned chickpeas, rinsed and drained
- 1/2 avocado, sliced
- 1/2 carrot, shredded
- 2 tablespoons tahini
- 1 tablespoon lemon juice
- Salt and pepper to taste

Step-by-Step Instructions

1. Start with a layer of brown rice or quinoa at the base of a bowl.

2. Add fresh spinach, chickpeas, avocado, and shredded carrot.

3. Whisk tahini, lemon juice, salt, and pepper together to make a dressing.

4. Drizzle the tahini dressing over the bowl and serve.

Nutritional Information per Serving

- Calories: 400
- Protein: 15g
- Carbohydrates: 55g
- Fat: 18g
- Fiber: 12g

Tips and Tricks

- Customize your Buddha bowl with your favorite veggies or protein.
- Prepare the ingredients in advance for an easy, quick lunch.

Grilled Portobello Mushroom Sandwich

A satisfying plant-based sandwich featuring juicy, umami-rich Portobello mushrooms. This recipe offers a hearty alternative to meat while incorporating fresh toppings for extra flavor.

Ingredients

- 2 large Portobello mushrooms, stems removed
- 2 whole grain sandwich buns
- 1/2 cup spinach
- 1/4 cup low-fat feta cheese (optional)
- 2 tablespoons balsamic vinegar
- Olive oil spray
- Salt and pepper to taste

Step-by-Step Instructions

1. Preheat a grill or grill pan over medium heat.
2. Brush the mushrooms with balsamic vinegar, a little olive oil, salt, and pepper.
3. Grill the mushrooms for about 5-7 minutes on each side until tender.

4. Assemble the sandwiches by placing the grilled mushrooms on the buns and adding spinach and feta, if desired.

5. Serve warm.

<u>Nutritional Information per Serving</u>

- Calories: 350
- Protein: 14g
- Carbohydrates: 45g
- Fat: 10g
- Fiber: 5g

<u>Tips and Tricks</u>

- Pair this sandwich with a side salad to make a more filling meal.
- You can also add toppings like hummus or roasted peppers for added flavor.

<u>Zucchini Noodles with Pesto</u>

Zucchini noodles with pesto provide a nutritious and refreshing twist on classic pasta dishes. The fresh basil pesto adds a burst of flavor, while the zucchini noodles offer a light, low-carb base—perfect for a healthy, satisfying lunch.

Ingredients

- 2 medium zucchinis, spiralized into noodles
- 1 cup fresh basil leaves
- 1/4 cup pine nuts
- 1/4 cup extra virgin olive oil
- 2 cloves garlic
- Salt and pepper to taste
- 2 tablespoons grated Parmesan cheese (optional)

Step-by-Step Instructions

1. In a food processor, blend together the basil, pine nuts, garlic, olive oil, salt, and pepper until smooth.
2. Heat a skillet over medium heat and add the zucchini noodles. Sauté for 2-3 minutes until they begin to soften slightly.
3. Remove from heat and toss the zucchini noodles with the pesto until well combined.
4. Serve immediately and top with grated Parmesan if desired.

Nutritional Information per Serving

- Calories: 240

- Protein: 5g
- Carbohydrates: 8g
- Fat: 22g
- Fiber: 3g

Tips and Tricks:

- Be careful not to overcook the zucchini noodles as they can quickly become too soft.
- Substitute sunflower seeds for pine nuts if you have a nut allergy.
- Add cherry tomatoes for extra flavor and color.

Sweet Potato and Black Bean Tacos

These colorful tacos are rich in fiber and plant-based protein, making them a great option for a satisfying lunch. The natural sweetness of the sweet potatoes combines beautifully with the heartiness of black beans, creating a delicious meal.

Ingredients

- 1 medium sweet potato, peeled and diced
- 1 can (15 oz) black beans, rinsed and drained
- 1 tablespoon olive oil

- 1 teaspoon cumin
- 1/2 teaspoon smoked paprika
- Salt and pepper to taste
- 4 corn tortillas
- Fresh cilantro, chopped (for garnish)
- Lime wedges (for serving)

Step-by-Step Instructions

1. Preheat your oven to 425°F (220°C).

2. Toss the diced sweet potato in a bowl with olive oil, cumin, smoked paprika, salt, and pepper until well coated.

3. Spread the sweet potato evenly on a baking sheet and roast for about 25-30 minutes, or until tender and slightly caramelized.

4. Heat the black beans in a saucepan over medium heat until warmed through.

5. Assemble the tacos by placing a portion of roasted sweet potatoes and black beans on each corn tortilla.

6. Top with fresh cilantro and serve with lime wedges.

Nutritional Information per Serving (2 tacos)

- Calories: 350
- Protein: 12g
- Fat: 8g
- Carbohydrates: 62g
- Fiber: 12g
- Sodium: 210mg

Tips and Tricks

- Customize your tacos with toppings like avocado, salsa, or shredded lettuce.
- Prepare extra sweet potatoes to use in salads or wraps later in the week.
- For a spicy kick, add diced jalapeños or a drizzle of hot sauce.

Brown Rice Sushi Rolls with Avocado

These sushi rolls offer a fun and nutritious way to enjoy a balanced lunch. With healthy fats from avocado and fiber from brown rice, they are both satisfying and tasty.

Ingredients

- 1 cup cooked brown rice

- 4 sheets of nori (seaweed)
- 1 ripe avocado, sliced
- 1 cucumber, julienned
- 1 carrot, julienned
- Soy sauce (low-sodium) for dipping

Step-by-Step Instructions

1. Lay a sheet of nori on a bamboo sushi mat or a clean surface.
2. Wet your hands to prevent sticking, and spread about 1/4 cup of cooked brown rice evenly over the nori, leaving a 1-inch border at the top.
3. Place slices of avocado, cucumber, and carrot in a line across the rice.
4. Starting from the bottom, roll the sushi tightly away from you, using the mat to help shape it.
5. Seal the edge of the nori with a little water.
6. Repeat with the remaining ingredients.
7. Slice the rolls into bite-sized pieces and serve with low-sodium soy sauce.

Nutritional Information per Serving (2 rolls)

- Calories: 300
- Protein: 6g

- Fat: 12g
- Carbohydrates: 42g
- Fiber: 10g
- Sodium: 250mg

Tips and Tricks
- Experiment with additional fillings like bell peppers, sprouts, or cooked shrimp.
- Serve with pickled ginger and wasabi for a traditional touch, keeping sodium levels in mind.
- Make extra rice for grain bowls or stir-fries later in the week.

Roasted Beet and Walnut Salad

This vibrant salad is not only visually striking but also rich in antioxidants, healthy fats, and essential nutrients. The earthy flavor of roasted beets pairs wonderfully with crunchy walnuts and fresh greens.

Ingredients
- 2 medium beets, roasted and sliced
- 2 cups mixed salad greens
- 1/4 cup walnuts, toasted

- 1/4 cup feta cheese, crumbled (optional)
- 2 tablespoons balsamic vinaigrette

Step-by-Step Instructions

1. Preheat your oven to 400°F (200°C).

2. Wrap each beet in foil and roast for 45-60 minutes, or until tender. Allow to cool, then peel and slice.

3. In a large bowl, mix the salad greens, roasted beets, and toasted walnuts.

4. Drizzle with balsamic vinaigrette and gently toss to combine.

5. Top with crumbled feta cheese if desired.

Nutritional Information per Serving

- Calories: 250
- Protein: 8g
- Fat: 16g
- Carbohydrates: 22g
- Fiber: 6g
- Sodium: 180mg

<u>**Tips and Tricks**</u>

- Roast extra beets to use in sandwiches or grain bowls.
- Add a protein source like grilled chicken or chickpeas for a more substantial meal.
- Prepare the salad ahead of time but keep the dressing separate until serving to prevent wilting.

Mediterranean Quinoa Bowl

This quinoa bowl features a delightful combination of Mediterranean flavors, offering a nutritious mix of proteins, healthy fats, and vegetables. It's ideal for meal prep since it can be enjoyed warm or cold.

<u>**Ingredients**</u>

- 1 cup cooked quinoa
- 1/2 cup cherry tomatoes, halved
- 1/2 cup cucumber, diced
- 1/4 cup red onion, finely chopped
- 1/4 cup olives, sliced
- 2 tablespoons olive oil
- 1 tablespoon lemon juice
- Salt and pepper to taste

Step-by-Step Instructions

1. In a large bowl, combine the cooked quinoa, cherry tomatoes, cucumber, red onion, and olives.

2. In a small bowl, whisk together the olive oil, lemon juice, salt, and pepper.

3. Drizzle the dressing over the quinoa mixture and toss until well mixed.

4. Serve immediately or refrigerate for later use.

Nutritional Information per Serving

- Calories: 280
- Protein: 8g
- Fat: 14g
- Carbohydrates: 32g
- Fiber: 5g
- Sodium: 210mg

Tips and Tricks

- Add feta cheese or chickpeas for extra protein.
- Customize the vegetables according to your preferences or what you have on hand.

- This bowl is perfect for meal prep; store it in airtight containers in the fridge.

Chapter 5

Soothing Dinners for Relaxation and Relief

Living with Meniere's disease can be draining, making a nourishing and comforting dinner the perfect way to end your day. This chapter offers a variety of satisfying, low-sodium dinner recipes designed to calm both your body and mind as you unwind. Each dish is made with ingredients that promote your overall health while providing the cozy, comforting feeling you crave after a long day. By adding these meals to your routine, you can nourish your body, encourage relaxation, and help manage Meniere's symptoms effectively.

Baked Salmon with Fresh Herbs and Lemon

This baked salmon dish is light, refreshing, and full of flavor, thanks to fresh herbs and lemon. Rich in omega-3 fatty acids, salmon helps reduce inflammation and supports overall health, making it ideal for those managing Meniere's symptoms.

Ingredients

- 4 salmon fillets
- 2 tablespoons olive oil
- Juice of 1 lemon
- 2 cloves garlic, minced
- Fresh rosemary, thyme, and dill (1 tablespoon each)
- Black pepper to taste
- Lemon slices for garnish

Step by Step Instructions

1. Preheat oven to 375°F (190°C).
2. Place salmon fillets on a baking sheet lined with parchment paper.
3. In a small bowl, mix olive oil, lemon juice, garlic, and herbs.

4. Drizzle herb mixture over the salmon and season with black pepper.

5. Top each fillet with a lemon slice and bake for 15-20 minutes, or until salmon flakes easily.

Nutritional Information per Serving

- Calories: 280
- Protein: 25g
- Fat: 18g
- Carbohydrates: 3g
- Fiber: 1g
- Sodium: 50mg

Tips and Tricks

- Feel free to swap the herbs for basil or parsley based on your preference.
- Serve with steamed veggies or brown rice for a well-rounded meal.
- Cover with foil while baking to retain moisture.

Low-Sodium Vegetable Stir-Fry with Tofu

This colorful vegetable stir-fry with tofu is a balanced one-pan dish, perfect for a low-sodium diet. It is packed with fiber, protein, and nutrients, while still being gentle on the body. The low-sodium soy sauce or coconut aminos keeps the flavor intact without compromising on health.

Ingredients

- 1 block extra-firm tofu, drained and cubed
- 1 tablespoon olive oil
- 1 bell pepper, sliced
- 1 carrot, julienned
- 1 cup broccoli florets
- 1 cup snap peas
- 1/4 cup low-sodium soy sauce or coconut aminos
- 2 tablespoons rice vinegar
- 1 tablespoon honey or maple syrup
- 1 teaspoon grated ginger
- 2 cloves garlic, minced
- Black pepper to taste

Step by Step Instructions

1. Heat olive oil in a skillet over medium-high heat, cook tofu until browned. Set aside.

2. Add bell pepper, carrot, broccoli, and snap peas to the skillet, and stir-fry for 4-5 minutes.

3. Mix soy sauce, rice vinegar, honey, ginger, and garlic in a bowl.

4. Return tofu to skillet, add the sauce, and cook until heated through.

5. Sprinkle with black pepper before serving.

Nutritional Information per Serving

- Calories: 230
- Protein: 12g
- Fat: 12g
- Carbohydrates: 20g
- Fiber: 4g
- Sodium: 100mg

Tips and Tricks

- Use whatever veggies you have on hand, like mushrooms or zucchini.
- Serve over brown rice or quinoa for extra fiber.

- Pat tofu dry before cooking for a crispier texture.

Brown Rice and Mushroom Risotto

This mushroom risotto is hearty, satisfying, and perfect for a comforting dinner. Made with nutrient-rich brown rice, this dish delivers fiber, while the mushrooms provide a savory umami flavor, making it indulgent yet healthy.

Ingredients

- 1 tablespoon olive oil
- 1 onion, finely chopped
- 2 cloves garlic, minced
- 1 1/2 cups brown rice
- 5 cups low-sodium vegetable broth
- 2 cups sliced mushrooms
- 1/2 cup grated Parmesan cheese (optional)
- Fresh thyme for garnish
- Black pepper to taste

Step by Step Instructions

1. Heat olive oil in a saucepan, cook onion until soft.

2. Add garlic and brown rice, stirring to coat rice well.

3. Add vegetable broth gradually, one cup at a time, stirring frequently.

4. In a separate skillet, sauté mushrooms until tender.

5. Once rice is tender and creamy, stir in mushrooms and Parmesan cheese.

6. Season with black pepper and garnish with thyme.

Nutritional Information per Serving

- Calories: 310
- Protein: 10g
- Fat: 8g
- Carbohydrates: 50g
- Fiber: 4g
- Sodium: 90mg

Tips and Tricks

- For a vegan version, skip the cheese or use nutritional yeast.
- Keep stirring the risotto to get a creamy consistency.

- Add a splash of white wine for extra flavor.

Balsamic Glazed Chicken with Steamed Vegetables

This balsamic glazed chicken with steamed vegetables is a simple and nourishing dinner that combines lean protein with an array of colorful vegetables. The balsamic glaze gives the chicken a slight sweetness, making it a delicious option for those looking to manage their symptoms without sacrificing taste.

Ingredients

- 4 boneless, skinless chicken breasts
- 1/4 cup balsamic vinegar
- 2 tablespoons honey
- 2 cloves garlic, minced
- 1 tablespoon olive oil
- Black pepper to taste
- 2 cups mixed steamed vegetables (broccoli, carrots, green beans)

<u>**Step by Step Instructions**</u>

1. Mix balsamic vinegar, honey, minced garlic, and olive oil in a small bowl.

2. Heat a skillet over medium heat, cook chicken until browned on both sides.

3. Pour balsamic mixture over chicken, reduce heat, and cook until chicken is done and glaze is thick.

4. Season with black pepper and serve with steamed vegetables.

<u>**Nutritional Information per Serving**</u>

- Calories: 290
- Protein: 30g
- Fat: 10g
- Carbohydrates: 18g
- Fiber: 3g
- Sodium: 70mg

<u>**Tips and Tricks**</u>

- Ensure the chicken is coated evenly for maximum flavor.
- Serve with brown rice or quinoa for added carbs.

- Add a sprig of rosemary to the glaze for extra aroma.

Herb-Crusted Baked Cod

Herb-crusted cod is a light yet flavorful dish that's rich in protein and omega-3 fatty acids. The fresh herbs provide a vibrant taste while keeping it low in sodium, making it perfect for an easy and healthy evening meal.

Ingredients

- 4 cod fillets
- 2 tablespoons olive oil
- 1 cup whole wheat breadcrumbs
- 2 tablespoons fresh parsley, chopped
- 1 tablespoon fresh dill, chopped
- 1 tablespoon fresh thyme, chopped
- Black pepper to taste
- Lemon wedges for garnish

Step by Step Instructions

1. Preheat oven to 400°F (200°C).

2. In a bowl, combine breadcrumbs, parsley, dill, thyme, and black pepper.

3. Brush cod fillets with olive oil and press into breadcrumb mixture to coat evenly.

4. Place on a baking sheet and bake for 15 minutes, or until golden brown and cooked through.

5. Serve with lemon wedges for added freshness.

Nutritional Information per Serving

- Calories: 240
- Protein: 26g
- Fat: 10g
- Carbohydrates: 15g
- Fiber: 2g
- Sodium: 70mg

Tips and Tricks

- Use panko breadcrumbs for a crunchier texture.
- Serve with steamed asparagus or roasted veggies.
- Add lemon zest to the breadcrumb mixture for extra citrusy flavor.

Lentil and Sweet Potato Stew

This comforting lentil and sweet potato stew is an excellent choice for a satisfying dinner. Rich in fiber, protein, and complex carbohydrates, it provides lasting energy and helps in managing Meniere's symptoms. With its warm, satisfying flavors, this one-pot meal nurtures both the body and soul.

Ingredients

- 1 tablespoon olive oil
- 1 onion, chopped
- 2 cloves garlic, minced
- 2 medium sweet potatoes, peeled and diced
- 1 cup dried lentils, rinsed
- 4 cups low-sodium vegetable broth
- 1 can diced tomatoes (no added salt)
- 1 teaspoon ground cumin
- 1 teaspoon smoked paprika
- Fresh cilantro for garnish
- Black pepper to taste

Step by Step Instructions

1. In a large pot, heat the olive oil over medium heat. Sauté the onion and garlic until they are soft and fragrant, about 5 minutes.

2. Add the diced sweet potatoes and lentils, mixing well.

3. Pour in the vegetable broth and add the diced tomatoes along with their juices.

4. Stir in the cumin and smoked paprika. Bring the mixture to a boil.

5. Once boiling, reduce the heat to low, cover, and let it simmer for about 25-30 minutes, or until the lentils and sweet potatoes are tender.

6. Season with black pepper to taste and garnish with fresh cilantro before serving.

Nutritional Information per Serving

- Calories: 320
- Protein: 12g
- Fat: 6g
- Carbohydrates: 55g
- Fiber: 14g
- Sodium: 90mg

<u>**Tips and Tricks**</u>

- For added creaminess, stir in a splash of coconut milk just before serving.
- This stew can be prepared in advance and kept in the fridge for up to 4 days, making it perfect for meal prep.
- Toss in some spinach or kale during the last 5 minutes of cooking for a boost of greens.

Quinoa Stuffed Bell Peppers

Quinoa stuffed bell peppers are vibrant and nutritious, packed with protein, fiber, and essential vitamins. They serve as a filling and flavorful dinner option that can be prepared in advance and baked when you're ready to eat.

<u>**Ingredients**</u>

- 4 large bell peppers (any color)
- 1 cup cooked quinoa
- 1 can (15 oz) black beans, rinsed and drained
- 1 cup corn (fresh, frozen, or canned)
- 1 cup diced tomatoes (fresh or canned)
- 1 teaspoon cumin
- 1 teaspoon chili powder

- 1/2 teaspoon garlic powder
- Salt and pepper to taste
- Fresh cilantro for garnish (optional)

<u>Step by step instructions</u>

1. Preheat the oven to 375°F (190°C).

2. Cut the tops off the bell peppers and remove the seeds and membranes.

3. In a large bowl, mix the cooked quinoa, black beans, corn, diced tomatoes, cumin, chili powder, garlic powder, salt, and pepper.

4. Fill each bell pepper with the quinoa mixture, packing it gently.

5. Stand the stuffed peppers upright in a baking dish.

6. Cover the dish with aluminum foil and bake for 25-30 minutes.

7. Remove the foil and bake for an additional 10-15 minutes until the peppers are tender.

8. If desired, garnish with fresh cilantro and serve warm.

<u>**Nutritional information per serving (1 stuffed pepper)**</u>

- Calories: 220
- Protein: 10g
- Carbohydrates: 38g
- Dietary Fiber: 10g
- Total Fat: 3g
- Sodium: 190mg

<u>**Tips and Tricks**</u>

- Personalize the filling by adding your favorite vegetables or spices for extra flavor.
- Prepare these stuffed peppers in advance and store them in the refrigerator for up to three days before baking.
- Leftovers can be frozen for a quick meal later on.

<u>Spinach and Mushroom Lasagna</u>

This spinach and mushroom lasagna is a hearty and delicious option that's both comforting and nutritious. It's an excellent way to incorporate greens into your diet while enjoying classic lasagna flavors.

<u>**Ingredients**</u>

- 9 whole wheat lasagna noodles
- 2 cups fresh spinach, chopped
- 1 cup mushrooms, sliced
- 2 cups ricotta cheese (low-fat)
- 1 cup mozzarella cheese, shredded (part-skim)
- 1 jar (24 oz) marinara sauce (low sodium)
- 1 teaspoon Italian seasoning
- 1/2 teaspoon garlic powder
- Salt and pepper to taste

<u>**Step by step instructions**</u>

1. Preheat the oven to 375°F (190°C).

2. Cook the lasagna noodles according to the package instructions, then drain and set aside.

3. In a skillet over medium heat, sauté the mushrooms until tender, about 5 minutes.

4. Add the spinach to the skillet and cook until wilted, about 2 minutes.

5. In a large bowl, combine the ricotta cheese, Italian seasoning, garlic powder, salt, and pepper.

6. Spread a thin layer of marinara sauce in a 9x13 inch baking dish.

7. Layer three lasagna noodles over the sauce, followed by half of the ricotta mixture, half of the spinach and mushroom mixture, and a third of the mozzarella cheese.

8. Repeat the layers: noodles, remaining ricotta, remaining spinach and mushrooms, and another layer of noodles topped with the remaining marinara sauce and mozzarella cheese.

9. Cover with foil and bake for 30 minutes. Remove the foil and bake for an additional 15 minutes until the cheese is bubbly and golden.

Nutritional information per serving (1/6 of the recipe)

- Calories: 350
- Protein: 21g
- Carbohydrates: 40g
- Dietary Fiber: 4g
- Total Fat: 12g
- Sodium: 300mg

<u>**Tips and Tricks**</u>

- Add other vegetables like zucchini or bell peppers for additional nutrition.
- Leftover lasagna can be kept in the refrigerator for up to 4 days and also freezes well.

Grilled Zucchini and Eggplant Skewers

These grilled zucchini and eggplant skewers are a tasty, low-calorie choice perfect for a summer evening. They're easy to prepare and make a great side dish or main course when paired with your favorite grains.

<u>**Ingredients**</u>

- 2 medium zucchinis, sliced into thick rounds
- 1 large eggplant, cut into cubes
- 1 red bell pepper, cut into squares
- 1 yellow bell pepper, cut into squares
- 3 tablespoons olive oil
- 2 teaspoons balsamic vinegar
- 1 teaspoon garlic powder
- Salt and pepper to taste
- Fresh basil for garnish (optional)

<u>**Step by step instructions**</u>

1. Preheat your grill to medium-high heat.

2. In a large bowl, mix the olive oil, balsamic vinegar, garlic powder, salt, and pepper.

3. Add the zucchini, eggplant, and bell peppers to the bowl, tossing to coat.

4. Thread the vegetables onto skewers, alternating between zucchini, eggplant, and bell peppers.

5. Place the skewers on the grill and cook for 8-10 minutes, turning occasionally until the vegetables are tender and slightly charred.

6. Remove from the grill and garnish with fresh basil if desired.

<u>**Nutritional information per serving (2 skewers)**</u>

- Calories: 150
- Protein: 3g
- Carbohydrates: 12g
- Dietary Fiber: 4g
- Total Fat: 10g
- Sodium: 120mg

Tips and Tricks

- Marinate the vegetables for an hour before grilling for enhanced flavor.
- Serve these skewers with a side of quinoa or brown rice for a complete meal.

Chickpea and Cauliflower Curry

This chickpea and cauliflower curry is a filling dish brimming with flavor and nourishment. The combination of chickpeas and cauliflower offers a good source of protein and fiber while keeping the meal light and satisfying.

Ingredients

- 1 can (15 oz) chickpeas, rinsed and drained
- 1 small head of cauliflower, cut into florets
- 1 can (14 oz) light coconut milk
- 1 onion, diced
- 2 cloves garlic, minced
- 1 tablespoon curry powder
- 1 teaspoon ginger, grated
- 1 tablespoon olive oil
- Salt and pepper to taste
- Fresh cilantro for garnish (optional)

Step by step instructions

1. In a large pot, heat the olive oil over medium heat. Add the onion and garlic and sauté until the onion is translucent.

2. Stir in the curry powder and ginger, cooking for an additional minute.

3. Add the cauliflower florets and chickpeas, stirring to coat them with the spices.

4. Pour in the coconut milk and bring to a simmer.

5. Lower the heat and cover, cooking for 15-20 minutes until the cauliflower is tender.

6. Season with salt and pepper to taste and garnish with fresh cilantro before serving.

Nutritional information per serving (1 cup)

- Calories: 280
- Protein: 10g
- Carbohydrates: 30g
- Dietary Fiber: 8g
- Total Fat: 14g
- Sodium: 200mg

<u>**Tips and Tricks**</u>

- Serve the curry over brown rice or quinoa for a complete meal.
- This dish tastes even better the next day, making it great for leftovers!

Chapter 6

Symptom-Soothing Snacks and Sides

Nutrient-rich snacks and side dishes play an important role in managing Meniere's disease, helping you stay energized while being mindful of your symptoms. These often-overlooked additions to your diet can greatly support your wellbeing and keep cravings at bay between meals. In this chapter, you'll find a variety of easy, tasty snacks and sides that are low in sodium and packed with essential nutrients.

Whether you need a quick bite at home or something on the go, each recipe is crafted to be simple to make and gentle on your body. With an emphasis on fresh, wholesome ingredients, these options not only satisfy hunger but also support your health.

Including these nourishing snacks and sides in your daily routine can help you manage symptoms effectively while enjoying diverse flavors and textures. Explore these delightful recipes designed to keep you feeling balanced and satisfied all day long.

Low-Sodium Hummus with Cucumber Slices

This low-sodium hummus is a creamy and flavorful dip that pairs beautifully with crisp cucumber slices. It's not only satisfying but also rich in protein and fiber, making it an energizing snack.

Ingredients

- 1 can (15 oz) chickpeas, drained and rinsed
- 2 tablespoons tahini
- 2 tablespoons olive oil
- 2 tablespoons lemon juice
- 1 clove garlic, minced
- 1 teaspoon ground cumin
- 1/4 teaspoon paprika
- Fresh cucumbers, sliced

Instructions

1. In a food processor, combine chickpeas, tahini, olive oil, lemon juice, garlic, cumin, and paprika.
2. Blend until smooth, adding water to achieve your desired consistency.
3. Taste and adjust seasoning as needed.
4. Transfer to a serving bowl, garnish with olive oil drizzle and a sprinkle of paprika.
5. Serve with cucumber slices for dipping.

Nutritional Information (per serving, 2 tablespoons of hummus)

- Calories: 70
- Protein: 2g
- Total Fat: 4g
- Carbohydrates: 8g
- Fiber: 2g
- Sodium: 10mg

Tips and Tricks

- For added flavor, consider mixing in roasted red peppers or fresh herbs like parsley or cilantro.

- Store in an airtight container in the fridge for up to one week.

Spiced Sweet Potato Wedges

These spiced sweet potato wedges offer a healthy alternative to traditional fries. Roasted to a golden perfection, they provide a delightful sweet and savory flavor, making for a satisfying snack or side dish. They're packed with vitamins and antioxidants, ideal for soothing symptoms.

Ingredients

- 2 medium sweet potatoes, cut into wedges
- 2 tablespoons olive oil
- 1 teaspoon paprika
- 1/2 teaspoon garlic powder
- 1/2 teaspoon black pepper
- 1/4 teaspoon cayenne pepper (optional)

Instructions

1. Preheat your oven to 425°F (220°C).
2. Toss the sweet potato wedges in a bowl with olive oil, paprika, garlic powder, black pepper, and cayenne (if using).

3. Spread the wedges in a single layer on a parchment-lined baking sheet.

4. Roast for 25-30 minutes, flipping halfway through, until golden and tender.

5. Serve warm with your preferred low-sodium dipping sauce.

Nutritional Information (per serving, about 4 wedges)

- Calories: 130
- Protein: 2g
- Total Fat: 5g
- Carbohydrates: 22g
- Fiber: 3g
- Sodium: 20mg

Tips and Tricks

- For extra crispiness, soak the sweet potato wedges in water for 30 minutes prior to baking.
- Feel free to experiment with different spices, such as cinnamon or cumin, for unique flavors.

Quinoa-Stuffed Bell Peppers

These quinoa-stuffed bell peppers are a colorful and nutritious option. Packed with protein and fiber, they make for a hearty snack or side dish. This recipe can be enjoyed warm or cold, making it versatile for any occasion.

Ingredients

- 4 bell peppers (any color)
- 1 cup cooked quinoa
- 1/2 cup black beans, rinsed and drained
- 1/2 cup corn kernels (fresh or frozen)
- 1/2 teaspoon cumin
- 1/2 teaspoon chili powder
- Fresh cilantro, chopped (for garnish)

Instructions

1. Preheat your oven to 375°F (190°C).

2. Cut off the tops of the bell peppers and remove the seeds.

3. In a mixing bowl, combine the cooked quinoa, black beans, corn, cumin, and chili powder.

4. Stuff each pepper with the quinoa mixture, packing it gently.

5. Place the stuffed peppers upright in a baking dish and cover with foil.

6. Bake for 30 minutes until the peppers are tender.

7. Garnish with fresh cilantro before serving.

<u>Nutritional Information (per stuffed pepper)</u>

- Calories: 150
- Protein: 5g
- Total Fat: 2g
- Carbohydrates: 30g
- Fiber: 7g
- Sodium: 5mg

<u>Tips and Tricks</u>

- Prepare these ahead of time and store them in the fridge for a quick snack option.
- Feel free to customize the filling with additional vegetables or grains.

<u>Roasted Chickpeas for Crunch</u>

Roasted chickpeas are a crunchy, protein-rich snack that's perfect for satisfying cravings without added sodium. They can be seasoned to your liking, making them a delicious and healthy option.

Ingredients

- 1 can (15 oz) chickpeas, drained and rinsed
- 1 tablespoon olive oil
- 1 teaspoon garlic powder
- 1 teaspoon smoked paprika
- 1/2 teaspoon cumin
- Pinch of salt (optional)

Instructions

1. Preheat your oven to 400°F (200°C).

2. Pat the chickpeas dry with a paper towel and place them in a bowl.

3. Drizzle with olive oil and toss with garlic powder, smoked paprika, cumin, and a pinch of salt.

4. Spread the chickpeas in a single layer on a baking sheet.

5. Roast for 25-30 minutes, shaking the pan halfway through until crispy.

6. Let them cool slightly before serving.

Nutritional Information (per serving, 1/4 cup)

- Calories: 120
- Protein: 6g

- Total Fat: 3g
- Carbohydrates: 20g
- Fiber: 5g
- Sodium: 5mg

Tips and Tricks
- Store leftovers in an airtight container for up to three days, but enjoy them quickly for the best crunch.
- Try different seasonings like curry powder or chili flakes for varied flavors.

Cucumber and Avocado Sushi Bites

These cucumber and avocado sushi bites are light and refreshing, requiring no cooking. They make for a quick snack and are filled with healthy fats and nutrients. This recipe is a fun way to sneak in more veggies while keeping sodium levels low.

Ingredients
- 1 large cucumber
- 1 ripe avocado
- 1 tablespoon lime juice
- 1/4 teaspoon sesame oil

- Optional toppings: sesame seeds, chopped green onions, or radish sprouts

Instructions

1. Slice the cucumber into 1/2-inch thick pieces.

2. In a bowl, mash the avocado with lime juice and sesame oil until creamy.

3. Top each cucumber slice with a spoonful of the avocado mixture.

4. Garnish with sesame seeds, green onions, or radish sprouts if desired.

5. Serve immediately for a refreshing snack.

Nutritional Information (per serving, 2 bites)

- Calories: 80
- Protein: 2g
- Total Fat: 6g
- Carbohydrates: 6g
- Fiber: 3g
- Sodium: 0mg

Tips and Tricks

- For an extra kick, sprinkle a little chili powder on the avocado before serving.

- These can be prepared ahead of time and stored in the fridge for a quick, grab-and-go option.

Baked Kale Chips

Baked kale chips offer a crunchy and nutritious alternative to conventional snacks. They're simple to prepare and can be flavored to suit your preferences. Kale is packed with vitamins A, C, and K, making these chips not only tasty but also beneficial for your overall health.

Ingredients

- 1 bunch of kale, with stems removed and leaves torn into bite-sized pieces
- 1 tablespoon olive oil
- 1/2 teaspoon garlic powder
- 1/2 teaspoon nutritional yeast (optional, for a cheesy taste)
- Pinch of salt (optional)

Instructions

1. Preheat the oven to 350°F (175°C).

2. In a large bowl, combine the kale leaves with olive oil, garlic powder, nutritional yeast, and a pinch of salt, ensuring they are well-coated.

3. Arrange the seasoned kale in a single layer on a parchment-lined baking sheet.

4. Bake for 10-15 minutes, flipping halfway through, until the chips are crisp but not burnt.

5. Allow them to cool before serving to preserve their crunchiness.

Nutritional Information (per serving, about 1 cup)

- Calories: 50
- Protein: 2g
- Total Fat: 4g
- Carbohydrates: 8g
- Fiber: 1g
- Sodium: 10mg (without added salt)

Tips and Tricks

- Feel free to try different spices, such as cayenne pepper or smoked paprika, for added flavor.

- For optimal crunch, enjoy the chips shortly after baking, as they may lose their crispness over time.

Carrot and Celery Sticks with Herb Dip

This colorful and crunchy snack features fresh vegetables paired with a flavorful herb dip, providing a refreshing option suitable for any time of day. Packed with vitamins and low in calories, it's an excellent choice for managing your symptoms.

Ingredients

- 2 large carrots, cut into sticks
- 2 celery stalks, cut into sticks
- 1 cup Greek yogurt (or a dairy-free alternative)
- 1 tablespoon fresh dill, chopped
- 1 tablespoon fresh parsley, chopped
- 1 teaspoon garlic powder
- Salt and pepper to taste (optional)

Step-by-step instructions

1. In a small bowl, mix together the Greek yogurt, dill, parsley, garlic powder, salt, and pepper until well combined.

2. Arrange the carrot and celery sticks on a platter.

3. Serve the herb dip alongside the vegetable sticks for dipping.

Nutritional information per serving (1/4 of dip recipe)

- Calories: 80
- Protein: 6g
- Carbohydrates: 10g
- Fat: 2g
- Sodium: 50mg

Tips and Tricks

- You can use any fresh herbs you like, such as chives or basil, as a substitute.
- For added flavor, consider adding a splash of lemon juice to the dip.

Apple Slices with Almond Butter

This easy and satisfying snack combines the sweetness of apples with the creamy texture of almond butter. It's not only tasty but also provides a substantial source of protein and fiber.

Ingredients

- 1 large apple (any variety), sliced
- 2 tablespoons almond butter (or a nut-free alternative)

Step-by-step instructions

1. Core the apple and slice it into thin wedges.
2. Arrange the apple slices on a plate and drizzle or scoop almond butter over the top.

Nutritional information per serving

- Calories: 180
- Protein: 4g
- Carbohydrates: 24g
- Fat: 9g
- Sodium: 1mg

<u>**Tips and Tricks**</u>
- For an extra treat, sprinkle cinnamon on the apple slices before serving.
- To prevent browning, toss the apple slices in a bit of lemon juice.

Steamed Edamame with Lemon

These lightly steamed edamame pods are not only enjoyable to eat but also provide a great source of protein. The zesty lemon adds a refreshing kick, making it a perfect snack option at any time.

<u>**Ingredients**</u>
- 1 cup frozen edamame pods (in shells)
- 1 tablespoon fresh lemon juice
- Sea salt to taste (optional)

<u>**Step-by-step instructions**</u>
1. Bring a pot of water to a boil and add the edamame pods.
2. Steam for about 3-5 minutes until tender yet still bright green.
3. Drain the edamame and place them in a bowl.

4. Drizzle with lemon juice and sprinkle with sea salt if desired.

Nutritional information per serving

- Calories: 120
- Protein: 10g
- Carbohydrates: 10g
- Fat: 5g
- Sodium: 0mg (without added salt)

Tips and Tricks

- Add a pinch of red pepper flakes for a spicy kick.
- Store any leftovers in an airtight container in the refrigerator for up to three days.

Mixed Nuts and Seed Trail Mix

This energizing trail mix blends various nuts and seeds, providing a satisfying crunch along with healthy fats and proteins. It's perfect for snacking on the go or for a midday energy boost.

Ingredients

- 1/2 cup unsalted almonds

- 1/2 cup unsalted walnuts
- 1/2 cup pumpkin seeds
- 1/2 cup sunflower seeds
- 1/4 cup dried cranberries or raisins (optional)

Step-by-step instructions

1. In a large bowl, combine all the nuts, seeds, and dried fruit (if using).
2. Mix thoroughly and store in an airtight container.

Nutritional information per serving (1/4 cup)

- Calories: 200
- Protein: 7g
- Carbohydrates: 10g
- Fat: 18g
- Sodium: 0mg

Tips and Tricks

- Feel free to personalize your trail mix by adding your favorite seeds or other nuts.
- Portion out servings in small bags for convenient, on-the-go snacks.

Chapter 7

Tasty Desserts Without Excess Salt or Sugar

Desserts can still bring comfort and joy, even when managing Meniere's disease. This chapter provides a range of dessert recipes that are both delicious and mindful of your health needs. Each treat is crafted to be low in sodium and added sugars, so you can satisfy your sweet tooth without affecting your wellbeing. These recipes highlight the natural sweetness of fruits and other wholesome ingredients, offering a healthier way to enjoy dessert while supporting symptom relief.

Indulge in these desserts with the assurance that managing Meniere's doesn't mean missing out on a delightful treat. Let's dive into recipes that prioritize flavor and wellness while avoiding unnecessary salt and sugar.

Berry Chia Pudding

This berry chia pudding is a delicious, nutritious dessert loaded with fiber and antioxidants. The chia seeds add a delightful texture and are a fantastic source of omega-3 fatty acids, making this pudding a guilt-free treat.

Ingredients

- 1 cup unsweetened almond milk (or any plant-based milk)
- 1/4 cup chia seeds
- 1 cup mixed berries (fresh or frozen)
- 1 teaspoon vanilla extract
- Optional: 1 tablespoon maple syrup or honey (if desired for extra sweetness)

Step-by-step instructions

1. In a bowl, whisk together the almond milk, chia seeds, vanilla extract, and sweetener (if using).

2. Mix well to eliminate any clumps of chia seeds.

3. Cover the bowl and refrigerate for at least 2 hours, or overnight, until thickened.

4. After setting, stir the pudding again to break up clumps.

5. Serve in individual bowls or jars topped with mixed berries.

Nutritional information per serving

- Calories: 160
- Protein: 5g
- Carbohydrates: 18g
- Dietary Fiber: 10g
- Total Sugars: 4g
- Fat: 7g

Tips and Tricks

- Try different types of milk for various flavors.
- Add a sprinkle of cinnamon or nutmeg for extra warmth.
- This pudding can also double as a nutritious breakfast option.

Fresh Fruit Salad with Lime Drizzle

A fresh fruit salad is a refreshing dessert that can be tailored with your favorite seasonal fruits. The lime drizzle adds a zesty twist, enhancing the fruits' natural sweetness.

Ingredients

- 2 cups mixed fresh fruit (e.g., watermelon, pineapple, strawberries, blueberries, kiwi)
- Juice of 1 lime
- Zest of 1 lime
- 1 tablespoon honey or agave syrup (optional)

Step-by-step instructions

1. In a large bowl, combine the chopped fresh fruit.
2. In a small bowl, mix lime juice, lime zest, and honey or agave syrup (if using).
3. Drizzle the lime dressing over the fruit and toss gently to combine.
4. Serve immediately, or chill for 30 minutes to enhance the flavors.

Nutritional information per serving

- Calories: 90

- Protein: 1g
- Carbohydrates: 22g
- Dietary Fiber: 2g
- Total Sugars: 15g
- Fat: 0g

Tips and Tricks

- Feel free to use any combination of fruits; aim for a variety of colors for visual appeal.
- For an added twist, include fresh mint leaves for extra freshness.

Banana Nice Cream

Banana nice cream is a quick, creamy dessert made by blending frozen bananas. It's an excellent substitute for ice cream, offering natural sweetness and a creamy texture without added sugars or dairy.

Ingredients

- 2 ripe bananas, sliced and frozen
- 1 tablespoon almond butter (or any nut butter)
- 1/2 teaspoon vanilla extract

- Optional toppings: sliced nuts, berries, or dark chocolate shavings

Step-by-step instructions

1. Place the frozen banana slices in a food processor.
2. Add almond butter and vanilla extract.
3. Blend until smooth and creamy, scraping the sides as needed.
4. Serve immediately for a soft-serve texture, or freeze for 30 minutes for a firmer consistency.
5. Add your preferred toppings before serving.

Nutritional information per serving

- Calories: 150
- Protein: 2g
- Carbohydrates: 25g
- Dietary Fiber: 3g
- Total Sugars: 12g
- Fat: 6g

Tips and Tricks

- Make sure the bananas are fully ripe for optimal sweetness.

- You can mix in other frozen fruits like mango or strawberries for different flavors.

<u>Baked Apples with Cinnamon</u>

These baked apples offer warmth and comfort, stuffed with oats, nuts, and cinnamon. They provide a satisfying end to your meal while being gentle on your digestive system.

<u>Ingredients</u>

- 4 medium apples (e.g., Granny Smith or Fuji)
- 1/2 cup rolled oats
- 1/4 cup chopped walnuts or pecans
- 1 teaspoon cinnamon
- 2 tablespoons maple syrup or honey
- 1 cup water

<u>Step-by-step instructions</u>

1. Preheat your oven to 350°F (175°C).

2. Core the apples and create a small cavity for stuffing.

3. In a bowl, mix the oats, nuts, cinnamon, and maple syrup.

4. Stuff the mixture into the cored apples.

5. Place the apples in a baking dish and pour water around them.

6. Cover with foil and bake for 25-30 minutes, or until the apples are tender.

<u>Nutritional information per serving</u>

- Calories: 180
- Protein: 3g
- Carbohydrates: 30g
- Dietary Fiber: 5g
- Total Sugars: 10g
- Fat: 6g

<u>Tips and Tricks</u>

- Serve warm with a dollop of yogurt or a scoop of banana nice cream for added creaminess.
- Feel free to experiment with spices like nutmeg or ginger for varied flavors.

Oatmeal Cookies with Dark Chocolate Chips

These oatmeal cookies are a delightful treat that combines wholesome oats with the rich taste of dark chocolate. They are low in sugar and can satisfy your sweet cravings without guilt.

Ingredients

- 1 cup rolled oats
- 1/2 cup whole wheat flour
- 1/2 teaspoon baking soda
- 1/2 teaspoon cinnamon
- 1/4 cup coconut oil, melted
- 1/4 cup maple syrup or honey
- 1/2 cup dark chocolate chips

Step-by-step instructions

1. Preheat your oven to 350°F (175°C) and line a baking sheet with parchment paper.
2. In a bowl, combine the oats, flour, baking soda, and cinnamon.
3. In another bowl, mix the melted coconut oil and maple syrup.

4. Combine the wet ingredients with the dry ingredients and stir until just blended.

5. Fold in the dark chocolate chips.

6. Drop spoonfuls of dough onto the baking sheet, spacing them apart.

7. Bake for 12-15 minutes, until the edges are golden.

Nutritional information per serving (1 cookie)

- Calories: 80
- Protein: 1g
- Carbohydrates: 10g
- Dietary Fiber: 1g
- Total Sugars: 4g
- Fat: 4g

Tips and Tricks

- Store cookies in an airtight container to keep them fresh.
- You can mix in nuts or dried fruit for added flavor.

Coconut Mango Rice Pudding

Coconut mango rice pudding is a creamy, tropical dessert that combines rich coconut flavor with the sweetness of ripe mangoes. It's an ideal dessert to enjoy when you crave something light yet satisfying.

Ingredients

- 1 cup cooked brown rice
- 1 can (13.5 oz) coconut milk
- 1/4 cup unsweetened shredded coconut
- 1/2 teaspoon vanilla extract
- 1 ripe mango, diced
- Optional: Fresh mint leaves for garnish

Step-by-step instructions

1. In a saucepan, combine the cooked rice, coconut milk, shredded coconut, and vanilla extract.
2. Cook over medium heat, stirring occasionally until heated through.
3. Remove from heat and let it cool slightly.
4. Stir in the diced mango.
5. Serve warm or chilled, garnished with fresh mint leaves if desired.

<u>**Nutritional information per serving**</u>

- Calories: 200
- Protein: 3g
- Carbohydrates: 30g
- Dietary Fiber: 2g
- Total Sugars: 10g
- Fat: 8g

<u>**Tips and Tricks**</u>

- This pudding can be stored in the refrigerator for up to 3 days.
- Feel free to substitute the mango with other fruits like pineapple or berries for a different twist.

<u>Avocado Chocolate Mousse</u>

This creamy avocado chocolate mousse is an excellent dessert choice when you're craving something indulgent yet packed with nutrients. Avocado gives a smooth texture and a boost of healthy fats, while cocoa powder provides a rich chocolate flavor—all without dairy or refined sugar.

Ingredients

- 2 ripe avocados
- 1/4 cup unsweetened cocoa powder
- 1/4 cup maple syrup
- 1/4 cup unsweetened almond milk
- 1 teaspoon vanilla extract

Step by step instructions

1. Cut the avocados in half, remove the pits, and scoop out the flesh into a blender or food processor.
2. Add the cocoa powder, maple syrup, almond milk, and vanilla extract.
3. Blend until the mixture is smooth and creamy, scraping down the sides as needed.
4. Divide into serving bowls and refrigerate for at least 30 minutes before serving.

Nutritional information per serving

- Calories: 180
- Fat: 11g
- Carbohydrates: 20g
- Protein: 2g
- Sodium: 15mg

Tips and Tricks

- Top with a few fresh raspberries or cocoa nibs for added flavor and texture.
- Adjust the sweetness by adding more or less maple syrup to suit your preference.

No-Bake Almond Date Energy Bites

These no-bake almond date energy bites are perfect for a quick and healthy sweet treat. The natural sweetness of dates pairs well with the nutty almonds, providing a balanced and nutritious way to satisfy your sugar cravings while getting fiber and healthy fats.

Ingredients

- 1 cup pitted Medjool dates
- 1 cup almonds
- 1/4 cup unsweetened shredded coconut
- 1 tablespoon chia seeds
- 1/2 teaspoon cinnamon

Step by step instructions

1. Combine the dates and almonds in a food processor, blending until a sticky dough forms.

2. Add shredded coconut, chia seeds, and cinnamon, and pulse until well combined.

3. Roll the mixture into small balls, about a tablespoon each.

4. Place the energy bites on a plate or tray and chill for at least 20 minutes before eating.

<u>Nutritional information per serving</u>

- Calories: 90
- Fat: 5g
- Carbohydrates: 10g
- Protein: 2g
- Sodium: 2mg

<u>Tips and Tricks</u>

- Store in an airtight container in the refrigerator for up to a week.
- Roll the bites in extra shredded coconut for added texture and visual appeal.

<u>Poached Pears with Ginger Syrup</u>

Poached pears with ginger syrup are a light, refined dessert that offers natural sweetness with a hint of spicy warmth from ginger. Pears are hydrating and rich in fiber, making this a healthy yet satisfying option to enjoy without guilt.

Ingredients

- 2 ripe but firm pears
- 2 cups water
- 2 tablespoons honey or maple syrup
- 1 tablespoon freshly grated ginger
- 1 teaspoon vanilla extract

Step by step instructions

1. Peel the pears, cut them in half, and remove the cores.

2. In a saucepan, mix the water, honey or maple syrup, grated ginger, and vanilla extract.

3. Submerge the pears in the liquid and bring to a gentle simmer.

4. Cook for 15-20 minutes, or until the pears are tender.

5. Remove the pears from the saucepan and let them cool slightly. Serve with a drizzle of the ginger syrup.

<u>**Nutritional information per serving**</u>

- Calories: 100
- Fat: 0.5g
- Carbohydrates: 25g
- Protein: 0.5g
- Sodium: 5mg

<u>**Tips and Tricks**</u>

- You can serve the pears warm or chilled, based on your preference.
- Garnish with a sprinkle of cinnamon or fresh mint leaves for extra flavor.

Raspberry Yogurt Parfait

This raspberry yogurt parfait is a refreshing and easy-to-make dessert that balances creamy yogurt with tart raspberries. It's an ideal way to end your meal on a light note. The yogurt provides protein while the raspberries add antioxidants, making it both nutritious and satisfying.

<u>**Ingredients**</u>

- 1 cup unsweetened plain Greek yogurt
- 1/2 cup fresh raspberries

- 2 tablespoons low-sugar granola
- 1 tablespoon honey (optional)

Step by step instructions

1. In a serving glass, layer yogurt, followed by raspberries.

2. Sprinkle one tablespoon of granola over the raspberries.

3. Repeat the layers, finishing with raspberries and a drizzle of honey if desired.

4. Serve immediately or chill until ready to enjoy.

Nutritional information per serving

- Calories: 150
- Fat: 5g
- Carbohydrates: 18g
- Protein: 9g
- Sodium: 60mg

Tips and Tricks

- To enhance the flavor, stir in a pinch of cinnamon into the yogurt.
- Feel free to use any other berries, like blueberries or strawberries, for variety.

Chapter 8

Hydration and Nourishing Beverages

Staying well-hydrated is key to managing Meniere's disease and greatly benefits your health and symptom control. Choosing the right beverages can help maintain hydration levels and support your body's balance. In this chapter, we introduce a selection of delicious drinks designed to be gentle on your system while enhancing your wellness.

Each recipe features low-sodium, nutrient-rich ingredients that help ease symptoms and encourage healthy hydration habits. From soothing herbal teas to revitalizing smoothies, these beverages will keep you refreshed and supply essential nutrients for better health.

Proper hydration plays a crucial role in reducing the frequency and intensity of vertigo episodes associated with Meniere's. By adding these simple, nourishing drinks to your daily routine, you can support inner ear health and overall vitality. Let's dive into these refreshing recipes that are as enjoyable as they are beneficial.

Herbal Teas for Inner Ear Health

Herbal teas provide a comforting and hydrating option that can offer various health benefits beneficial for managing Meniere's symptoms. This particular tea is made with herbs known for their anti-inflammatory properties.

Ingredients

- 1 tablespoon dried ginger root
- 1 tablespoon dried peppermint leaves
- 2 cups boiling water
- Honey (optional, for sweetness)

Step-by-step instructions

1. Combine the dried ginger and peppermint leaves in a teapot or heatproof container.

2. Pour boiling water over the herbs.

3. Cover and steep for 10 minutes.

4. Strain the tea into a cup and sweeten with honey if desired.

Nutritional information per serving

- Calories: 0 (without honey)
- Total Fat: 0g
- Sodium: 0mg
- Carbohydrates: 0g

Tips and Tricks

- Experiment with other herbs like chamomile or lemon balm for added health benefits.
- Enjoy this tea warm for soothing effects or cool it down and serve over ice for a refreshing drink.

Low-Sugar Berry Smoothie

This berry smoothie is a delightful way to hydrate while benefiting from the antioxidants in berries. It's naturally low in sugar and packed with vitamins.

Ingredients

- 1 cup mixed berries (strawberries, blueberries, raspberries)
- 1 banana
- 1 cup unsweetened almond milk
- 1 tablespoon chia seeds
- Ice cubes (optional)

Step-by-step instructions

1. In a blender, combine the mixed berries, banana, almond milk, and chia seeds.
2. Blend until smooth.
3. If desired, add ice cubes and blend again for a frosty texture.
4. Pour into a glass and enjoy!

Nutritional information per serving

- Calories: 150
- Total Fat: 5g
- Sodium: 115mg
- Carbohydrates: 25g
- Fiber: 5g

Tips and Tricks

- Substitute frozen fruit if fresh berries are unavailable.
- For a protein boost, add a scoop of plant-based protein powder.

Electrolyte Balancing Infused Water

Infused water is a refreshing way to stay hydrated while obtaining essential electrolytes. This simple recipe combines hydrating ingredients known for supporting bodily functions.

Ingredients

- 1 lemon, sliced
- 1 cucumber, sliced
- A handful of fresh mint leaves
- 2 liters of water

Step-by-step instructions

1. Combine lemon slices, cucumber, and mint leaves in a large pitcher.
2. Fill the pitcher with water and stir gently.
3. Allow it to infuse in the refrigerator for at least 2 hours before serving.

<u>**Nutritional information per serving**</u>

- Calories: 5
- Total Fat: 0g
- Sodium: 0mg
- Carbohydrates: 1g

<u>**Tips and Tricks**</u>

- Feel free to mix and match with other fruits and herbs, such as berries or basil.
- Keep a jug in your fridge to encourage regular hydration throughout the day.

Ginger Lemonade for Digestive Comfort

Ginger lemonade is not only refreshing but also has digestive benefits that can soothe your stomach while promoting hydration.

<u>**Ingredients**</u>

- 1 tablespoon fresh ginger, grated
- 1 lemon, juiced
- 2 cups water
- Honey (optional)

Step-by-step instructions

1. In a small saucepan, combine the grated ginger and water.

2. Bring to a boil and then let it simmer for 5 minutes.

3. Remove from heat, strain the ginger, and let the liquid cool.

4. Mix in the lemon juice and honey if using.

5. Serve over ice or chilled.

Nutritional information per serving

- Calories: 20 (without honey)
- Total Fat: 0g
- Sodium: 0mg
- Carbohydrates: 5g

Tips and Tricks

- Adjust the amount of lemon or ginger to suit your taste.
- This drink can be stored in the refrigerator for up to 3 days.

Cucumber and Mint Cooler

This refreshing cucumber and mint cooler is ideal for warm days, providing hydration while delivering a burst of flavor.

Ingredients

- 1 cucumber, peeled and diced
- A handful of fresh mint leaves
- 2 cups sparkling water
- Lime slices (for garnish)

Step-by-step instructions

1. In a blender, combine the diced cucumber and mint leaves.
2. Blend until smooth, then strain to remove pulp.
3. Pour the cucumber-mint juice into a glass.
4. Top with sparkling water and garnish with lime slices.

Nutritional information per serving

- Calories: 15
- Total Fat: 0g
- Sodium: 0mg
- Carbohydrates: 3g

<u>**Tips and Tricks**</u>
- For a twist, add a splash of fresh lime or lemon juice.
- This cooler can be prepared in larger batches and stored in the fridge.

Anti-Inflammatory Golden Milk

Golden milk is a comforting beverage made with turmeric, recognized for its anti-inflammatory properties. It's a soothing drink that can be enjoyed warm or chilled.

<u>**Ingredients**</u>
- 1 cup unsweetened almond milk
- 1 teaspoon turmeric powder
- 1/2 teaspoon cinnamon
- 1 teaspoon honey or maple syrup (optional)
- A pinch of black pepper

<u>**Step-by-step instructions**</u>

1. In a small saucepan, combine almond milk, turmeric, cinnamon, and black pepper.

2. Heat over medium until warm, stirring frequently.

3. Remove from heat and stir in honey or maple syrup if desired.

4. Pour into a cup and enjoy warm or allow it to cool for a refreshing cold drink.

Nutritional information per serving

- Calories: 40
- Total Fat: 2g
- Sodium: 0mg
- Carbohydrates: 6g

Tips and Tricks

- Add a dash of ginger for an extra kick.
- Golden milk can also be enjoyed before bedtime for its calming effects.

Watermelon Basil Cooler

This cooling drink combines the hydrating benefits of watermelon with the aromatic flavor of basil, providing a refreshing boost that helps combat fluid retention. Watermelon is packed with water and electrolytes, making this beverage an excellent choice for staying hydrated.

Ingredients

- 2 cups watermelon, cubed
- 4-5 fresh basil leaves
- 1 cup cold water
- Juice of 1/2 lemon
- Ice cubes (optional)

Step-by-Step Instructions

1. Add watermelon, basil leaves, cold water, and lemon juice to a blender.
2. Blend until smooth and combined well.
3. Strain if a smoother consistency is preferred.
4. Pour into a glass and add ice if desired.

Nutritional Information per Serving

- Calories: 50
- Carbohydrates: 13g
- Sugars: 10g
- Vitamin C: 15% of Daily Value (DV)
- Potassium: 6% of DV

<u>**Tips and Tricks**</u>
- Garnish with lemon slices or extra basil leaves for presentation.
- Add a teaspoon of honey for extra sweetness.
- Chill the watermelon before blending for a cooler beverage.

Green Detox Juice

This detox juice features hydrating ingredients like cucumber, apple, and spinach. It helps flush out toxins, reduces fluid retention, and delivers key nutrients that support ear health.

<u>**Ingredients**</u>
- 1 cucumber, chopped
- 1 green apple, cored and chopped
- 1 handful spinach
- Juice of 1/2 lemon
- 1 cup cold water

<u>**Step-by-Step Instructions**</u>
1. Blend the cucumber, apple, spinach, lemon juice, and cold water in a blender until smooth.

2. Strain through a fine mesh sieve for a juice-like consistency if desired.

3. Serve chilled.

<u>Nutritional Information per Serving</u>

- Calories: 70
- Carbohydrates: 17g
- Fiber: 3g
- Vitamin A: 20% of DV
- Vitamin C: 25% of DV

<u>Tips and Tricks</u>

- Add a small piece of ginger for extra flavor and digestive support.
- Mint leaves make a great addition for freshness.
- Drink immediately to retain all the nutrients.

<u>Blueberry Coconut Smoothie</u>

This creamy smoothie combines antioxidant-rich blueberries with hydrating coconut water. Blueberries help reduce inflammation, and coconut water adds a natural source of electrolytes to support proper hydration.

<u>**Ingredients**</u>

- 1 cup blueberries (fresh or frozen)
- 1/2 cup plain yogurt (dairy or non-dairy)
- 1/2 cup coconut water
- 1 tablespoon chia seeds
- Ice cubes (optional)

<u>**Step-by-Step Instructions**</u>

1. Add blueberries, yogurt, coconut water, and chia seeds to a blender.
2. Blend until smooth and creamy.
3. Pour into a glass and add ice if desired.

<u>**Nutritional Information per Serving**</u>

- Calories: 120
- Protein: 4g
- Carbohydrates: 18g
- Fiber: 4g
- Vitamin C: 20% of DV

<u>**Tips and Tricks**</u>

- Use frozen blueberries for a thicker smoothie without needing ice.

- For added protein, include a scoop of your favorite protein powder.
- Garnish with extra blueberries or chia seeds for a decorative touch.

Lemon Ginger Iced Tea

This iced tea blends the soothing properties of ginger with a zesty lemon flavor, creating a hydrating drink that helps manage Meniere's symptoms. Ginger helps reduce inflammation, and lemon provides a refreshing boost of vitamin C.

Ingredients
- 2 cups water
- 1-inch piece of fresh ginger, sliced
- Juice of 1 lemon
- 1 teaspoon honey (optional)
- Ice cubes

Step-by-Step Instructions
1. Bring water to a boil in a pot.
2. Add ginger slices and let it steep for about 10 minutes.
3. Remove from heat and allow the tea to cool.

4. Strain the ginger tea, then add lemon juice and honey if using.

5. Serve over ice.

<u>Nutritional Information per Serving</u>

- Calories: 20
- Carbohydrates: 6g
- Vitamin C: 15% of DV
- Sugar: 5g (with honey)

<u>Tips and Tricks</u>

- Prepare a larger batch to keep on hand in the refrigerator for easy access.
- Adjust the ginger to your taste preference—more ginger adds more spice.
- Add mint leaves for a cooling twist.

Integrating these hydrating beverages into your daily routine can significantly benefit your overall health and help ease Meniere's symptoms. From calming herbal teas that soothe to invigorating smoothies that energize, each drink offers a delicious way to nourish your body while enhancing hydration.

As you try out these recipes, keep in mind that proper hydration is a crucial component of your wellness journey. Make it a habit to choose these flavorful drinks throughout the day, and you'll not only enjoy their taste but also the supportive role they play in symptom management.

Embrace the variety of options in this chapter to discover your favorites. By prioritizing hydration and nutrition, you empower yourself to live more fully with Meniere's disease. Savor these beverages as delightful additions to your meals, contributing positively to your path toward improved wellbeing.

Chapter 9

Planning Meals for Meniere's Relief

Effective meal planning is essential in managing Meniere's disease symptoms. A well-structured plan supports a low-sodium diet and ensures you receive key nutrients needed for overall health. This 21-day meal plan offers a diverse selection of balanced meals that are gentle on the body and designed to help ease symptoms.

Weekly Meal Plan for Symptom Management

Week 1
Day 1

- **Breakfast:** Anti-Inflammatory Berry Smoothie Bowl

- **Lunch:** Roasted Veggie and Quinoa Salad
- **Dinner:** Baked Salmon with Fresh Herbs and Lemon
- **Snack:** Low-Sodium Hummus with Cucumber Slices

Day 2

- **Breakfast:** Quinoa Porridge with Fresh Berries
- **Lunch:** Lemon Herb Chicken Wraps
- **Dinner:** Low-Sodium Vegetable Stir-Fry with Tofu
- **Snack:** Spiced Sweet Potato Wedges

Day 3

- **Breakfast:** Low-Sodium Vegetable Omelette
- **Lunch:** Low-Sodium Lentil Soup
- **Dinner:** Brown Rice and Mushroom Risotto
- **Snack:** Quinoa-Stuffed Bell Peppers

Day 4

- **Breakfast:** Banana Oat Pancakes with No-Added-Sugar Syrup

- **Lunch:** Spinach and Chickpea Buddha Bowl
- **Dinner:** Balsamic Glazed Chicken with Steamed Vegetables
- **Snack:** Roasted Chickpeas for Crunch

Day 5

- **Breakfast:** Chia Seed Pudding with Almonds
- **Lunch:** Grilled Portobello Mushroom Sandwich
- **Dinner:** Herb-Crusted Baked Cod
- **Snack:** Cucumber and Avocado Sushi Bites

Day 6

- **Breakfast:** Avocado Toast with Lemon Zest
- **Lunch:** Zucchini Noodles with Pesto
- **Dinner:** Lentil and Sweet Potato Stew
- **Snack:** Baked Kale Chips

Day 7

- **Breakfast:** Overnight Oats with Apples and Cinnamon
- **Lunch:** Sweet Potato and Black Bean Tacos

- **Dinner:** Quinoa Stuffed Bell Peppers
- **Snack:** Carrot and Celery Sticks with Herb Dip

Week 2

Day 8

- **Breakfast:** Spinach and Mushroom Frittata
- **Lunch:** Brown Rice Sushi Rolls with Avocado
- **Dinner:** Spinach and Mushroom Lasagna
- **Snack:** Apple Slices with Almond Butter

Day 9

- **Breakfast:** Buckwheat Pancakes with Blueberries
- **Lunch:** Roasted Beet and Walnut Salad
- **Dinner:** Grilled Zucchini and Eggplant Skewers
- **Snack:** Steamed Edamame with Lemon

Day 10

- **Breakfast:** Ginger and Turmeric Smoothie

- **Lunch:** Mediterranean Quinoa Bowl
- **Dinner:** Chickpea and Cauliflower Curry
- **Snack:** Mixed Nuts and Seed Trail Mix

Day 11

- **Breakfast:** Anti-Inflammatory Berry Smoothie Bowl
- **Lunch:** Roasted Veggie and Quinoa Salad
- **Dinner:** Baked Salmon with Fresh Herbs and Lemon
- **Snack:** Low-Sodium Hummus with Cucumber Slices

Day 12

- **Breakfast:** Quinoa Porridge with Fresh Berries
- **Lunch:** Lemon Herb Chicken Wraps
- **Dinner:** Low-Sodium Vegetable Stir-Fry with Tofu
- **Snack:** Spiced Sweet Potato Wedges

Day 13

- **Breakfast:** Low-Sodium Vegetable Omelette
- **Lunch:** Low-Sodium Lentil Soup

- **Dinner:** Brown Rice and Mushroom Risotto
- **Snack:** Quinoa-Stuffed Bell Peppers

Day 14

- **Breakfast:** Banana Oat Pancakes with No-Added-Sugar Syrup
- **Lunch:** Spinach and Chickpea Buddha Bowl
- **Dinner:** Balsamic Glazed Chicken with Steamed Vegetables
- **Snack:** Roasted Chickpeas for Crunch

Week 3

Day 15

- **Breakfast:** Chia Seed Pudding with Almonds
- **Lunch:** Grilled Portobello Mushroom Sandwich
- **Dinner:** Herb-Crusted Baked Cod
- **Snack:** Cucumber and Avocado Sushi Bites

Day 16

- **Breakfast:** Avocado Toast with Lemon Zest
- **Lunch:** Zucchini Noodles with Pesto
- **Dinner:** Lentil and Sweet Potato Stew
- **Snack:** Baked Kale Chips

Day 17

- **Breakfast:** Overnight Oats with Apples and Cinnamon
- **Lunch:** Sweet Potato and Black Bean Tacos
- **Dinner:** Quinoa Stuffed Bell Peppers
- **Snack:** Carrot and Celery Sticks with Herb Dip

Day 18

- **Breakfast:** Spinach and Mushroom Frittata
- **Lunch:** Brown Rice Sushi Rolls with Avocado
- **Dinner:** Spinach and Mushroom Lasagna
- **Snack:** Apple Slices with Almond Butter

Day 19

- **Breakfast:** Buckwheat Pancakes with Blueberries

- **Lunch:** Roasted Beet and Walnut Salad
- **Dinner:** Grilled Zucchini and Eggplant Skewers
- **Snack:** Steamed Edamame with Lemon

Day 20

- **Breakfast:** Ginger and Turmeric Smoothie
- **Lunch:** Mediterranean Quinoa Bowl
- **Dinner:** Chickpea and Cauliflower Curry
- **Snack:** Mixed Nuts and Seed Trail Mix

Day 21

- **Breakfast:** Anti-Inflammatory Berry Smoothie Bowl
- **Lunch:** Roasted Veggie and Quinoa Salad
- **Dinner:** Baked Salmon with Fresh Herbs and Lemon
- **Snack:** Low-Sodium Hummus with Cucumber Slices

Tips for Meal Prep and Batch Cooking

1. **Plan Ahead:** Spend some time each week to map out your meals and create a grocery list based on the necessary ingredients.

2. **Batch Cooking:** Make larger quantities of soups, stews, and grains (like quinoa and brown rice) to use during the week. Store them in airtight containers for easy access.

3. **Utilize the Freezer:** Prepared meals can be frozen in single portions, providing a quick option when time is limited.

4. **Stay Flexible:** Feel free to adjust meals based on your preferences or available ingredients. The main goal is to keep meals low in sodium while enjoying a range of flavors.

5. **Incorporate Leftovers:** Plan meals that creatively use leftovers. For example, roasted vegetables from dinner can enhance a lunch salad.

Grocery Shopping List for a Low-Sodium Diet

- **Fruits:** Fresh berries, bananas, apples, lemons, sweet potatoes, avocados
- **Vegetables:** Spinach, kale, zucchini, bell peppers, cucumbers, mushrooms, carrots, beets, eggplant
- **Grains:** Quinoa, brown rice, buckwheat, whole-grain oats
- **Proteins:** Salmon, chicken breast, tofu, lentils, chickpeas, black beans, eggs
- **Nuts and Seeds:** Almonds, mixed nuts, chia seeds
- **Herbs and Spices:** Fresh herbs (parsley, cilantro, basil), turmeric, ginger, black pepper
- **Condiments:** Low-sodium soy sauce, balsamic vinegar, olive oil

This carefully crafted meal plan empowers you to take charge of your dietary choices while addressing the challenges of Meniere's disease. By focusing on nourishing, low-sodium meals, you are making significant strides toward easing symptoms and enhancing your overall health.

Chapter 10

Lifestyle Tips for Living Well with Meniere's

This chapter provides practical tips and strategies to help reduce stress, enhance sleep quality, stay physically active, and create a supportive environment that promotes a well-balanced lifestyle.

Stress Reduction Techniques

Managing stress effectively is crucial for individuals with Meniere's disease, as stress can intensify symptoms such as vertigo and tinnitus. Consider these beneficial strategies:

1. **Mindfulness and Meditation**
   - Practicing mindfulness helps ground you and alleviate anxiety. Set aside a few minutes daily for meditation, concentrating on your

breath and releasing negative thoughts. Consider using apps like Headspace or Calm for guided sessions.

2. **<u>Deep Breathing Exercises</u>**
   - Deep breathing can trigger the body's relaxation response. Inhale deeply through your nose for four counts, hold for four, and exhale slowly through your mouth for six counts. Repeat several times to promote calmness.

3. **<u>Yoga and Gentle Movement</u>**
   - Incorporating gentle yoga or stretching into your routine can enhance relaxation and flexibility. Look for classes or online resources tailored for individuals facing balance challenges.

4. **<u>Regular Breaks</u>**
   - If symptoms become overwhelming during the day, take regular breaks to rest and recharge. Even a few moments of quiet can significantly help.

5. <u>Journaling</u>

- Keeping a journal allows you to express your thoughts and feelings. Document your symptoms, emotions, and potential triggers, which can assist in discussions with your healthcare provider.

<u>The Importance of Sleep and Exercise</u>

Getting enough sleep and maintaining an active lifestyle are crucial for effective Meniere's disease management.

<u>*Sleep Hygiene*</u>

1. <u>Create a Relaxing Bedtime Routine</u>

- Develop a soothing pre-sleep routine with calming activities such as reading or taking a warm bath. Strive to go to bed and rise at the same time each day to establish a consistent sleep cycle.

2. **Optimize Your Sleep Environment**

- Make your bedroom sleep-friendly by keeping it dark, cool, and quiet. Consider blackout curtains, earplugs, or a white noise machine as needed.

3. **Limit Stimulants**

- Avoid caffeine and nicotine in the hours leading up to bedtime, as they can disrupt sleep. Additionally, limit screen time from devices like smartphones and TVs at least an hour before sleep.

Physical Activity

1. **Gentle Exercises**

- Engage in low-impact activities such as walking, swimming, or cycling. Aim for at least 30 minutes of moderate exercise most days to boost cardiovascular health and alleviate stress.

2. **<u>Balance and Coordination Training</u>**

- Include exercises that enhance balance and coordination, which can help mitigate Meniere's symptoms. Tai Chi or Pilates can be especially beneficial for improving stability.

3. **<u>Listen to Your Body</u>**

- Be mindful of your body's responses to physical activity. If you experience dizziness or fatigue, take a break or adjust your exercise routine as necessary.

<u>Creating a Supportive Environment for Wellbeing</u>

Cultivating a nurturing environment can greatly enhance your quality of life.

1. **<u>Connect with Support Groups</u>**

- Look for local or online support groups for individuals with Meniere's disease. Connecting with others who share similar experiences can provide valuable insights and emotional backing.

2. **<u>Educate Family and Friends</u>**

- Share information about Meniere's disease with your loved ones. Educating them about your condition will help create a supportive network that can assist you when needed.

3. **<u>Plan Social Activities Mindfully</u>**

- When attending social events, choose quieter settings that are less likely to trigger symptoms. Don't hesitate to take breaks or excuse yourself if you start feeling overwhelmed.

4. **<u>Set Realistic Goals</u>**

- Focus on establishing achievable health and lifestyle goals that consider your condition. Celebrate your progress, no matter how small, and be willing to adjust your expectations as necessary.

5. **<u>Consult with Professionals</u>**

- Collaborate with healthcare providers, nutritionists, or therapists who specialize in

Meniere's disease to create a personalized plan that suits your needs and lifestyle.

Incorporating these lifestyle strategies can significantly enhance your ability to manage Meniere's disease. By embracing stress-relief practices, prioritizing quality sleep and physical activity, and creating a supportive environment, you can build a balanced lifestyle that supports well-being and resilience. Remember, everyone's journey is different, so be patient and tailor these approaches to suit your unique needs. Embrace each small step you take and empower yourself to live a fulfilling life despite the challenges Meniere's may bring.

Chapter 11

Frequently Asked Questions

This chapter addresses common inquiries related to Meniere's disease and dietary changes. Gaining insight into these topics can help you effectively manage symptoms and enhance your overall health.

Common Questions About Meniere's and Diet

1. What is Meniere's Disease, and how does diet influence it?

Meniere's disease is a condition affecting the inner ear, leading to episodes of vertigo, hearing loss, tinnitus, and a sensation of fullness in the ear. Although the exact cause is not fully understood, certain dietary choices can aid in symptom management. Following a low-sodium diet can help reduce fluid retention and lower pressure in the inner ear, potentially decreasing the frequency and intensity of vertigo episodes.

2. What dietary practices are effective for managing Meniere's symptoms?

To effectively manage symptoms of Meniere's disease, consider the following dietary practices:

- **Embrace a Low-Sodium Diet:** Limiting salt intake can help minimize fluid accumulation in the inner ear.
- **Maintain Hydration:** Staying well-hydrated is important for fluid balance.
- **Limit Caffeine and Alcohol:** Both can lead to dehydration and may worsen symptoms.
- **Incorporate Anti-Inflammatory Foods:** Include fruits, vegetables, whole grains, and lean proteins to support overall health and reduce inflammation.

3. Which foods should I avoid?

Certain foods may trigger symptoms for some people. Common triggers include:

- Processed foods high in sodium

- Caffeinated drinks
- Alcoholic beverages
- Foods with high sugar and saturated fat content

It's vital to pay attention to your body's reactions and steer clear of any foods that seem to aggravate your symptoms.

4. How can I ensure adequate nutrient intake on a low-sodium diet?

To maintain nutritional balance on a low-sodium diet, focus on foods that are naturally low in sodium but rich in nutrients:

- **Fruits and Vegetables:** Fresh produce is typically low in sodium and packed with vitamins and minerals.
- **Whole Grains:** Choose options like quinoa, brown rice, and whole oats.
- **Lean Proteins:** Incorporate skinless poultry, fish, legumes, and tofu.
- **Healthy Fats:** Include avocados, nuts, and seeds, which provide essential fatty acids without excessive sodium.

Consulting with a registered dietitian can help you create customized meal plans that meet your nutritional requirements.

5. How can I modify recipes to suit my dietary needs?

To adapt recipes for a low-sodium diet, consider the following strategies:

- **Reduce Salt Usage:** Enhance flavors using herbs, spices, and citrus instead of salt.
- **Select Low-Sodium Alternatives:** Choose low-sodium versions of condiments and canned items.
- **Experiment with Ingredients:** Replace high-sodium components with fresh or frozen options.

Practical Tips for Recipe Adaptation

1. Read Nutrition Labels

When buying packaged foods, always check the nutrition labels for sodium content. Aim for products containing less than 140 mg of sodium per serving, which qualifies as low-sodium.

2. Prioritize Fresh Ingredients

Using fresh ingredients gives you control over sodium levels and enhances meal flavor.

3. Utilize Flavor Enhancers

Incorporate vinegar, lemon juice, or various spices to add zest to your meals without adding salt.

4. Batch Cooking and Freezing

Preparing meals in larger quantities can save time and help you adhere to your dietary objectives. Freezing portions for busy days offers convenient meal options.

5. Keep a Food Journal

Maintaining a food diary can help track what you eat and how it affects your symptoms, allowing you to identify patterns and make better dietary choices.

Conclusion

Living with Meniere's disease may feel overwhelming at times, but with the right approach and tools, a balanced and fulfilling life is within reach. This book is crafted not only to provide you with enjoyable recipes tailored to Meniere's needs, but also to offer practical strategies for managing symptoms and simplifying daily routines. By focusing on nutrient-rich, low-sodium meals and hydrating drinks, you're actively working to ease vertigo, tinnitus, and other common symptoms.

Yet, nutrition is just one piece of the puzzle. Adopting healthy sleep routines, managing stress, staying physically active, and creating a supportive environment are all essential for achieving the best outcomes. The recipes and meal plans in this book are designed to help reduce symptom frequency and intensity while bringing joy to your meals.

Now is the time to move forward with confidence. Continue to explore new flavors, savor the comfort of wholesome meals, and embrace lifestyle changes that nurture your well-being. Remember, you're not alone on this path—there are resources, support groups, and communities to guide you.

By prioritizing self-care, listening to your body, and making thoughtful food choices, you're taking control of Meniere's rather than letting it control you. Embrace this new lifestyle and continue your journey toward improved health, one meal at a time.